How

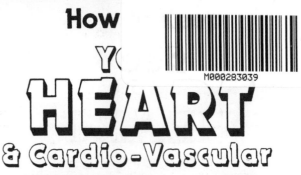

YOUR HEART
& Cardio-Vascular
HEALTHY and FIT
At Any Age

By
PAUL C. BRAGG, N.D., Ph.D.
LIFE EXTENSION SPECIALIST
and
PATRICIA BRAGG, Ph.D.
Health & Fitness Expert

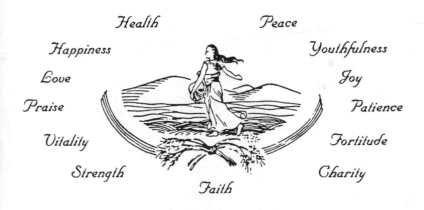

Health   *Peace*

Happiness   *Youthfulness*

Love   *Joy*

Praise   *Patience*

Vitality   *Fortitude*

Strength   *Charity*

Faith

JOIN

**The Bragg Crusades for a 100% Healthy, Vigorous,
Strong America and a Better World for All!**

HEALTH SCIENCE
Box 7, Santa Barbara, California 93102 U.S.A.

How To Keep
YOUR
HEART
& Cardio-Vascular
HEALTHY and FIT
At Any Age

By

PAUL C. BRAGG, N.D., Ph.D.
LIFE EXTENSION SPECIALIST

and

PATRICIA BRAGG, N.D., Ph.D.
LIFE EXTENSION NUTRITIONIST

- REVISED -
Copyright © Health Science

Fourteenth printing MCMXCII
ISBN: 0-87790-050-7

Published in the United States by
HEALTH SCIENCE - Box 7, Santa Barbara, Calif. 93102, USA

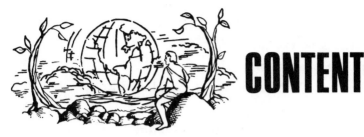

CONTENTS

From the Bragg home to your home we share our years of health knowledge—years of living close to God and Nature and what joys of fruitful, radiant living this produces—this my Father and I share with you and your loved ones.

Patricia Bragg

Contents

Contents

Contents

*52% of American's living today will die from cardiovascular disease–don't
be one of them–no excuses–start your healthy heart program today!*

Contents

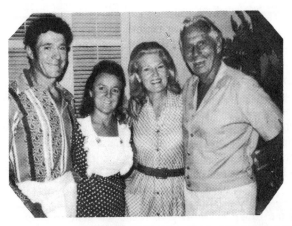

Jack LaLanne, Patricia Bragg, Elaine LaLanne & Paul Bragg

Jack says, "Bragg saved my life at age 14 when I attended the Bragg Health & Fitness Lecture in Oakland, California." From that day on, Jack has lived the health life and teaches Health & Fitness to millions.

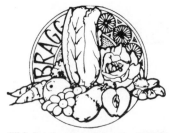

FROM THE AUTHORS

This book was written for YOU. It can be your passport to the Good Life. We Professional Nutritionists join hands in one common objective - high standard of health for all and many added years to your life. Scientific Nutrition points the way - Nature's Way - the only lasting way to build a body free of degenerative diseases and premature aging. This book teaches you how to work with Nature and not against her. Doctors, dentists and others who care for the sick try to repair depleted tissues, which too often mend poorly - if at all. Many of them praise the spreading of this new scientific message of natural foods and methods for long-lasting health and youthfulness at any age. To speed the spreading of this tremendous message, this book was written.

Statements in this book are recitals of scientific findings, known facts of physiology, biological therapeutics and reference to ancient writings as they are found. Paul C. Bragg has been practicing the natural methods of living for over 80 years with highly beneficial results, knowing they are safe and of great value. His daughter Patricia Bragg works with him to carry on the Health Crusade. They make no claims as to what the methods cited in this book will do to one in any given situation, and assume no obligation because of opinions expressed.

No cure for disease is offered in this book. No foods or diets are offered for the treatment or cure of any specific ailment. Nor is it intended as, or to be used as, literature for any food product. Paul C. Bragg and Patricia Bragg express their opinions solely as Public Health Educators, Professional Nutritionists and Teachers.

Certain persons considered experts may disagree with one or more statements in this book, as the same relate to various nutritional recommendations. However, any such statements are considered, nevertheless, to be factual, as based upon long-time experience of Paul C. Bragg and Patricia Bragg in the field of human health.

BRAGG BLESSINGS FROM OUR HOME

From the Bragg home to your home we share our years of health knowledge-years of living close to God and Nature and what joys of fruitful, radiant living this produces-this my Father and I share with you and your loved ones. With Blessing for Health and Happiness,

Patricia Bragg

*Dear friend, I wish above all things that thou may prosper
and be in health even as the soul prospers* - 3 John 2

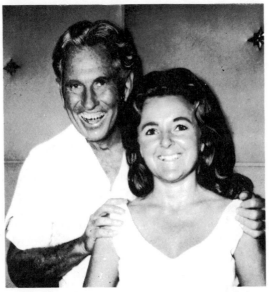

Paul C. Bragg and daughter, Patricia

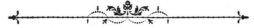

WHY WE WROTE THIS BOOK:

Cardiovascular (heart and blood vessel) problems constitute the No. 1 Killer in the civilized world today. Yet these problems can be prevented and controlled! Thousands of our health students throughout the world have developed ... strong hearts from weak hearts...averted bypass heart surgery, rejuvenated their circulatory systems...by following the methods of Natural Living and Natural Eating outlined in this book.

My father, Paul C. Bragg ... pioneered these precepts and practiced them for almost a century...with an "ageless" heart in a biologically youthful body even as a great-great-grandfather! We have both thrived on a Diet of Natural Foods all our lives...no salt, no refined white sugar or flour, no artificial additives or poisonous preservatives, no debilitating drinks. . . only natural "live" foods. . . combined with a Program of Healthful Exercise, Relaxation and Revitalizing Sleep.

We want to share with you the knowledge we have gained from experience and research. . . so that you, too, may no longer dread the No. 1 Killer ... but become and remain truly Young in Heart for the rest of your life !

Only 20% of American's have some form of regular exercise!
This is causing poor health and mounting cardiovascular
disease. A regular exercise program is important for heart
health – Start your daily exercise program today.

HEALTHY HEART HABITS FOR A LONG VITAL LIFE

Remember, you are what you eat, drink & do, so eat a low-fat, low-sugar, high-fiber diet of natural whole grains and starches, fresh salad greens, sprouts, vegetables, garlic, fresh fruits, raw seeds, nuts, pure juices and distilled water (chemical free).

Earn your food with daily exercise, for regular exercise improves your health, stamina, flexibility, endurance, & helps open up the cardiovascular system. Only 45 minutes a day can do miracles for your mind and body.

We are made of tubes. To help keep them clean & open, make a mixture using 2/3 raw oat bran and 1/3 psyllium husk powder and add 2-3 tablespoons daily to juices, pep drinks, herbal teas, soups, hot cereals, etc. Be sure that it's wet and expanded for 2 minutes.

Niacin (B-3) helps also to cleanse and open the cardiovascular system. Take regular-released Niacin (100mg) with one meal daily. After cholesterol level reaches 180 or lower, you can take Niacin once or twice weekly.

Remember, your heart needs a good balance of nutrients, so take a natural vitamin-mineral food supplement with extra vitamin (mixed Tocopherols), the new Ester-C, Magnesium and Beta Carotene, for these are your heart's super helpers!

Also use this amazing enzyme SOD (super oxide dismutase) for it helps flush out dangerous free radicals that can cause havoc with your cardiovascular pipes and general health. Latest research shows extra benefits...promotes longevity, slows aging & fights arthritis & its stiffness, swelling & pain, and it helps prevent jet lag exhaustion and cataracts.

Count your blessings daily while you do your brisk walking and exercises with these affirmations – "health! strength! youth! vitality! peace! laughter! humbleness! energy! understanding! forgiveness! joy! and love!"– and soon all these qualities will come flooding and bouncing into your life.

Healthy Fiber Habit: Make a mixture of two-thirds raw oat bran and one-third psyllium husk powder and use 3-5 tablespoons a day in juices, soups, herbal teas, pep drinks, cereals, muffins, etc., plus ample salads, fresh fruits, vegetables, legumes and 100% whole grains! Fiber helps reduce cholesterol, varicose veins and helps normalize blood pressures. Fiber helps keep you regular and reduce hemorrhoids and is a natural body weight normalizer.

To maintain good health the body must be exercised properly (walking, jogging, running, biking, swimming, deep breathing, good posture, etc.) and nourished wisely (natural foods), so as to provide and increase the good life of radiant health, joy and happiness. —Paul C. Bragg

How to Keep the Heart Healthy and Fit

MY ACTIVE, BUSY LIFE TODAY

As a Nutritionist I travel over the world, teaching the principles of Scientific Nutrition to thousands of health-conscious students. Every year I personally interview and give Nutritional-Fitness Programs to some 7,000 people. Among my outstanding students in Nutrition are leading personalities of the film industry, TV and radio, as well as opera, ballet and concert artistes.

I also supervise a vast acreage of certified and guaranteed organically-grown foods, and conduct exhaustive research projects on plant, animal and human nutrition. My working day averages 12 hours. I have a painless, tireless, ageless body.

I WAS A "BLUE BABY"

This robust health which I enjoy today was acquired by the methods which I shall explain in this book. I was born with a weak heart—a "blue baby"—on a plantation deep in the heart of Virginia, where large quantities of tobacco and peanuts were grown and hogs were raised. Even in the modern hospitals of today a "blue baby" has to fight for its life.

During the first fourteen months of my life there was a constant struggle to survive. From infancy I suffered severe attacks of heart palpitation. At eight years of age I was stricken with rheumatic fever, and for eleven days hovered between life and death.

My weak heart prevented me from engaging in the activities of a normal, healthy country boy. Along with this weak heart I developed other physical weaknesses . . . sinusitus, asthma and bronchitis. Finally, in my teens, I came down with tuberculosis. I spent several years in large sanatoriums in Denver and Lake Saranac, where death sentences were pronounced upon me. There seemed to be no hope for my survival.

FROM DEGENERATION TO REJUVENATION

But where there is life there is hope. I was miraculously inspired to go to a famous sanatorium in Switzerland. And it was there that the famous Dr. Rollier, who is known as the "AIR, WATER, SUNSHINE, EXERCISE AND GOOD NUTRITION" DOCTOR, used natural methods and restored my broken body to buoyant, radiant health.

In a short period of time I rebuilt my body and started my climb toward super-strength and energy!

Another important event happened in my life at this time . . . I made the greatest decision of my life for my future. I decided to *devote my life to helping others to find* the treasure I had found . . . *Priceless Radiant Health!* Yes, that was the channel into which I wanted to direct the wonderful new energy and vitality I had found. So many persons are searching blindly for "the light"—how to find health. I had found the magic formula of Natural Living . . . now I desired to pass on this great message to others so that they, too, would be led from the darkness of sickness into the crystal clear light and brilliance of Super-Health!

For a number of decades I have been researching along these same Natural Methods . . . and have given this message to many thousands of people all over the world. My files are filled with almost unbelievable testimonials of what Natural Methods will do to rebuild the heart and body.

I now lay before you a Plan of Living based on Natural Laws . . . it can do for you what it has done for me.

THE WORLD'S MOST WONDERFUL MACHINE—YOUR BODY

Suppose a magician suddenly appeared before you and promised you a marvelous machine which could run itself, direct itself, repair itself, perform remarkable mental and physical feats . . . and would last for about 120 years and then some. Would you treasure such a machine? Of course you would! You would keep it in top condition in order to obtain a

---

Having heard the word, keep it, and bring forth fruit with patience. —Luke 8:15

maximum of service. Every day you would be astonished anew by the performance of this miracle-machine!

True, this is an age of mechanical marvels ... but remember that the supreme tribute we can pay to any machine is to say, "It is almost human."

Now stop and think! The Creator has presented you with the world's most wonderful machine—YOUR OWN BODY. This miracle-machine has its own *non-stop motor* (the heart), its own *fueling system* (the digestive tract), its own *filtration system* (kidneys), its own *thinking apparatus* (brain and nervous system), its own *temperature controls* (sweat glands), etc. Indeed, this most remarkable contrivance even has the *power to reproduce* itself!

KEEP THIS MACHINE FUNCTIONING AT PEAK EFFICIENCY

And yet, until illness strikes, how do you take care of your body? By "care" I do not mean "coddling." I mean those sensible practices and precautions which keep us in trim for the vigorous workaday routine that strenuous modern living requires.

Most people are lucky enough to be born healthy, but far too often take this priceless gift for granted ... and unfortunately, Nature does not always let them get away with this carefree attitude. You can ruin a good car by neglect or abuse ... and you can do exactly the same with a good constitution.

Unless you know how your body functions—or mis-functions—you cannot take proper care of it. Most people's ideas about their physical processes are erroneous or far-fetched. Even in this scientific age, too many superstitions and old wives' tales about the human body still persist.

In this book you will find set forth the complete story of HOW THE BODY WORKS, together with a straight forward account of the mental and emotional factors which influence it. There will also be valuable suggestions as to how to keep your system running at peak efficiency!

The book that will benefit most is the one that inspires men to think and to act for themselves. —Elbert Hubbard

DON'T BLAME HEART ATTACK ON HARD WORK—
STRESS—STRAIN—TENSION

You hear so much about the modern "rat race" today. You hear people telling you that the great pleasures of our "mile a minute" pace of living cause the heart attacks. The words "hard work" . . . "stress" . . . "strain" . . . "tension" . . . are used as excuses for the rising death rates from heart attacks.

The basis for the heart attack is coronary blockage. The blockage grows silently, insidiously. There is no way of knowing how much rust is accumulating inside the arteries until it is too late. The question is often asked, "Is there no warning before the blood supply to the heart begins to get dangerously low?"

In some parts of the body, such as the legs, a reduced blood supply to the muscles can cause localized pain sensations. But *in the heart itself there are no nerves which can specifically localize pain.* This is why so many flabby people, who eat any rubbish set before them, will tell you that they are in fine shape without special care of the body. But when they have the heart attack, do they ever blame it on their own rotten habits of living? Oh, no!—it was the hard work, pressures and tensions they were under.

Let's get the record straight. Since the dawn of history humans have lived under tremendous pressures, stress, strain and tension. That is exactly what life is—pressures. To live and exist each 24 hours means bearing up under pressures of all kinds. Man as we know him never lived without pressures.

PRIMITIVE MAN LIVED UNDER GREAT PRESSURES

Our primitive ancestors lived under pressures which would be difficult for us to survive. Primitive man was the prey of wild animals hunting to kill and eat him. His fellow humans were also hunting to kill him. Tribes and even families were constantly warring with one another. Wind, rain, snow and bad weather of all kinds put him under severe pressure. He had to survive against cruel and vicious natural forces such as floods, tornadoes, earthquakes, hurricanes . . . plagues, famines, epidemics.

4

Man has evolved under great pressures of all kinds. Stress, strain and tension are nothing new to humanity.

I believe that man can face the hardest pressures that life can put upon him, if he is strong of body and alert of mind. It is the survival of the fittest.

Heart trouble is not an inevitable attendant upon the mounting hard work, stress, strain, tension and pressures that modern people face daily.

People of the past had to exist under tremendous pressures. But they were rugged people, active physically and mentally. Their secret was good, substantial, natural food with an abundance of physical activity and exercise.

THE SECRET OF SURVIVAL

As in the past, so it is today. Build yourself a vigorous, strong body and you can face the great pressures that are part of our culture today. Health, strength, endurance, stamina, vitality and energy are your weapons against pressures, stresses, strains and tensions.

Let's face the facts. This is a tough, rough, cruel and hardboiled world we live in today. And woe to the weak for they shall perish!

Self Preservation is the First Law of Life. And that's what this book is all about. You who find yourself here on earth . . . YOU must get fit for the battle of life. And there is no substitute for life.

It's up to you, whether you're rich or poor, to fight for your continued health with exercise and proper eating.

DON'T LOSE YOUR HEALTH TO GAIN WEALTH

I regard as basically unintelligent the man or woman who sits back and makes money for 15 or 20 years while they allow their health to slip . . . and then when they get a heart attack or some other crippling ailment say, "I have worked so hard . . . I have been under terrible pressures and tensions. All my troubles are due to these strains."

Tell me what you eat and I will tell you what you are. — **Paul C. Bragg**

Poppycock! Had they given proper attention to their physical bodies they could have made their money and still enjoyed perfect health.

Hundreds of times we hear wealthy people say, *"I'd give all my wealth for my health."* If they had applied a combination of commonsense and a little effort, *they could have had both.* All that is needed is an elementary knowledge of the working of the body and its basic needs, and the sense to recognize abuses and how to avoid them.

Most people spend years mastering their careers ... but wouldn't spend five minutes attempting to learn anything about the limitations and needs of the body. Yet health is essential for the full enjoyment over a long life of the improved financial conditions which they are so intent upon creating.

YOU CAN COME BACK PHYSICALLY

One of the most remarkable things about the human body is its ability to repair itself. If you cut yourself, for example, the cells will heal and in time the wound and the scar will be replaced by new tissue. If you break a bone, it will knit after it has been set and become as strong as ever. Unexpected injury may come to anyone ... but if you have been taking care of your body, the chances are that you will recover quickly and with a minimum of discomfort.

Less obvious injuries that have accumulated over a period of time may also be repaired by the amazing human body. After taking a hammering for years, after being totally neglected for far too long, *your body can make recoveries far greater than you realize* ... if you're prepared to put in the time and effort and observe a little patience. Just as a business that has been allowed to slip can be rebuilt ... so can a neglected body.

But don't expect an overnight miracle. It takes a person a long time to break the body down ... and it takes time to rebuild it.

The human body has one ability not possessed by any machine— the ability to repair itself. —George E. Crile, Jr., M.D.

FOR AN AGELESS HEART—
AN OUNCE OF PREVENTION IS WORTH A TON OF CURE

Living by the principles of proper diet and plenty of exercise is the Royal Road to Health and Long Life.

Most people wait until something disastrous happens in the body before they do anything. In this Natural Program for Fitness that I am giving you, I will teach the Prevention System of taking care of the body.

You can have an ageless and a powerful heart at any age!

You can start today and rebuild not only your heart, but your entire body.

We obtain most of our energy from the food we eat, which has been directly and indirectly acted upon by the rays of the sun. Therefore, *diet* is of the greatest important in the maintenance of health.

The next is that we must keep the blood circulating over the great pipe system of the body. This is done by *exercise* and physical activity.

The results will be worth all the effort you put into this work. You will be rewarded with a powerful heart and a strong body that can take any pressures put upon you. In fact, you will welcome challenges. No matter how big or how serious the problem . . . with your powerful body you can face with a smile the worst that life can offer you.

HEART ATTACK—THE NO. 1 KILLER

Diseases of the heart and blood vessels take more than 1 million American lives each year . . . more than all other causes of death combined! In addition to being the No. 1 Killer, it is also the No. 1 Health Destroyer. More than 22 million people in the United States—of all ages—suffer from some form of heart trouble or disease of the blood vessels. Those who survive one heart attack live in constant dread of another.

The chances are better than 2-to-1 that—directly or indirectly—the adult male American will die of some heart disease. 92,000,000 Americans living today will eventually die of heart disease—*unless they start a Prevention Program.*

Clinical studies recently reported by The American Heart Association show that we are almost at the point where—through proper diet and exercise—a healthy heart can be virtually guaranteed. Unfortunately, this truly exciting news received relatively minor newspaper coverage and aroused too little interest. Keeping people well does not make big headlines. Newsmen have a saying, "Great news is not interesting news." It is the sensational and the disastrous that make the headlines.

HEALTH IS YOUR WEALTH

Health, like freedom and peace, endures as long as we exert ourselves to maintain it.

It's almost exclusively in your hands whether you enjoy a healthy, vigorous life to a ripe old age . . . or whether you succumb to the slovenly, non-energetic existence and probable premature breakdown of health which happens to most people living in countries with what is known as "a high standard of living." In these countries coronary (heart) disease is the biggest killer. The "high standard of living" is not producing a "high standard of life."

In my opinion, the rising epidemic of *coronary disease is totally unnecessary*. It would not exist if people were educated to eat and exercise properly . . . if people would only realize that they have the power in their own hands—and feet —to protect themselves right through life.

I believe that most men and women go through life never knowing what it is to be really physically fit. They never know that vigorous feeling of well-being, the unlimited sources of energy and the moral boost of never being really tired. They miss out on achieving *the highest standard of living of all* . . . the greatest wealth—*health*!

ONE HEART, ONE LIFE

At birth, the majority of people are given a powerful heart. There are always exceptions, of course, like myself who was born a "blue baby" with a weak heart and had a hard fight to survive. But I did survive and I did develop an "ageless heart."

8

This marvelous heart that Nature gives us can go on beating indefinitely. Moses was 120 years old when he died; Noah was 950; Jared lived to be 962; and "all the days of Methuselah" were 969 years. Right here in the United States today we have more than 7,000 people who are 100 years or more. In my intense research on the study of long life I have met many men and women who were 120 to 130 years or more. It just shows that it is possible to live a long life ... and that as long as the heart beats you are alive. And what greater treasure is there than life!

I myself do not live by calendar years. I no longer celebrate birthdays. I live by biological or physical years. It doesn't really matter what your calendar age happens to be. In fact, it might be better all around to forget one's chronological age and consider only the anatomical or physiological age.

Longevity is really a vascular question. *"A man is as old as his arteries."* As Sir William Osler, the great Canadian Medical teacher and writer, pointed out long ago: "A man of twenty-eight-or-nine may have the arteries of a man of sixty, and a man of forty may present vessels as much degenerated as they could be at eighty ..."

Osler used this word *"degenerated."* Webster defines degeneration as: *"Deterioration of a tissue or an organ in which its vitality is diminished; a process by which normal tissue becomes converted into or replaced by tissue of inferior quality, either by chemical change of the tissue (true degeneration) or the deposit of abnormal matter in the tissue (infiltration)."*

We are given a heart with clean arteries when we are born. It is our vicious habits of living that bring on degeneration.

The care we take of our heart determines the number of years we are going to stay on top of this earth. It is up to each and every one of us to take special care of our heart so we can make this life a long, healthy and happy one. When you are healthy you are happy!

Of all the knowledge, that most worth having is knowledge about health. The first requisite of a good life is to be a healthy person. —Herbert Spencer

9

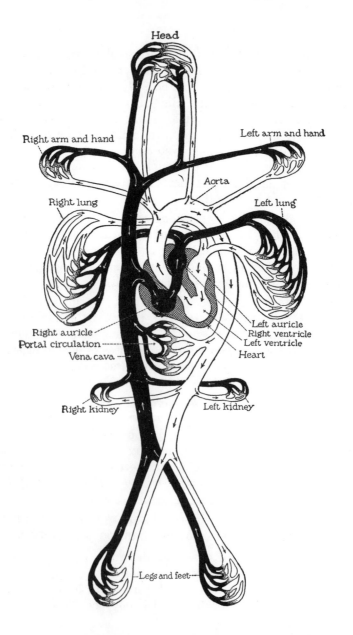

THE HEART AND BLOOD-VESSEL SYSTEM. The diagram shows the cycle from right heart through the lungs, to the left heart, then through the system back to the right heart. Note that all the blood from the digestive system goes through the portal veins; i.e., through the liver.

10

THE HEART AND THE CIRCULATORY SYSTEM

To understand the problems of heart trouble, we must know something about the heart and the circulatory system. The function of this intricate cardio-vascular (heart and blood vessels) system is to distribute blood throughout the entire body, bringing a steady flow of nourishment and oxygen to the billions of body cells, and removing toxic wastes from the cells.

The blood circulates in a network of *100,000 miles of blood vessels* that reach every cell in the body, from those of the heart itself to the top of the scalp and the tips of the fingers and toes. In the average individual there are from *six to eight quarts of blood circulating* in this vast network.

During rest or inactivity the blood makes one round trip per minute. During activity or exercise it may make as many as eight or nine round trips per minute, in order to supply the necessary fuel for the increased energy and remove the burnt-out wastes. Even during rest *the heart pumps* the prodigious amount of *13 tons of blood every 24-hour period.*

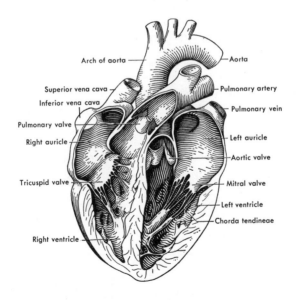

Arch of aorta — — Aorta

Superior vena cava — — Pulmonary artery
Inferior vena cava — — Pulmonary vein

Pulmonary valve — — Left auricle
Right auricle — — Aortic valve

Tricuspid valve — — Mitral valve
— Left ventricle
— Chorda tendineae

Right ventricle —

The heart is really a double pump, each side composed of two chambers, an auricle and a ventricle.

11

THE HEART IS A MUSCLE

The heart is not an organ of the body. It is a muscle—and a very powerful one. It has to be! You can readily see that the heart must be powerful and efficient to do all this work. Yet it is not much larger than your fist.

The heart is a muscular pump, whose vital task is to pump the blood and keep it circulating in a never-ending journey throughout the body. The tissues of the body—including the heart—need oxygen to spark the chemical reaction which provides energy, just as a fire needs oxygen before it will burn and generate heat. The blood's important function is to carry that oxygen to the tissues, as well as the food which provides the fuel.

The oxygen is first picked up from the air in the lungs. This oxygen-enriched blood (reddish in color) then travels to the heart and is pumped to the tissues where the oxygen content is given off. Blood depleted of oxygen is bluish in color, and returns to the heart to be pumped back into the lungs.

Thus the heart is receiving two types of blood simultaneously —oxygen-enriched blood from the lungs and the oxygen-depleted blood from the tissues.

To keep these two streams apart, the heart chamber is divided in two by a muscular partition called the septum. The left and right chambers formed by the septum are each divided into two compartments. One is the auricle, which has a thin wall, has little pumping action and serves mainly as a reservoir. The other is the ventricle which has a thick, muscular wall and does the main pumping.

When you have been stricken by illness, your new car, your new home, your new big bank balance—all these fade into unimportance until you have regained your vigor and zest for living again.
— Peter J. Steincrohn, M.D.

If your food is devitalized, the important elements of nourishment have been removed, or if its value has been diminished by wrong cooking processes—you can then starve to death on a full stomach.

The unexamined life is not worth living. It is a time to re-evaluate your past as a guide to your future. —Socrates

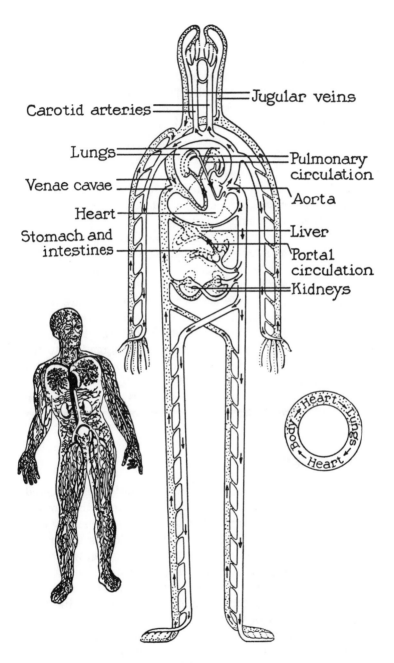

Diagram showing the circulation of the blood in the body.

INTRICATE NETWORK OF ARTERIES AND VEINS

The object of the circulation of the blood is to ensure that all the cells of the body shall be regularly supplied with food and oxygen, and regularly cleared of toxic substances. To achieve this objective an intricate network of tubes run throughout the body. These are the blood vessels.

The blood vessels which carry the blood *from the heart* are known as *arteries*. Those which *return the blood* to the heart are called *veins*. Both vary greatly in size, just like the streamlets and brooks and creeks which flow into a river, which may then join a larger river.

The *largest* blood vessel is the main artery, the *Aorta*, which is the main supply pipe leading directly out of the heart and from which—through numerous branches—all parts of the body are eventually supplied with blood.

The *smallest* of both the arteries and the veins are called *capillaries*—so tiny that most are only visible under a microscope. It is through these capillaries that the last of the food and oxygen is given off and the transfer is made into the veins, which carry the oxygen-depleted blood and toxic wastes back to the heart for purification. Enroute to the heart most of the wastes are transferred to the kidneys for elimination from the body through the urine. The carbon dioxide, another impurity, is expelled through the lungs.

BLOOD PURIFICATION

When the blood, which is now full of impurities collected from the tissues of the body, is returned to the heart through the veins, it is at once pumped out through a large artery into the lungs. There the blood gives off the last of its impurities (carbon dioxide) and absorbs the life-giving oxygen which the lungs have breathed in. (Please don't contaminate it with tobacco smoke!) The blood is then returned to the heart and is once more pumped out through the Aorta on its long journey to every part of the body.

Blood circulation is not simple. It follows a main design which resembles the figure 8. *There are actually two separate circulations—away from and back to the heart*. One, the

14

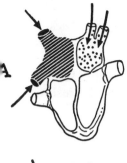

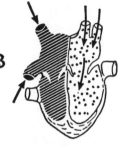

The flow of blood through the heart. The heart cycle, shown here in its four stages, takes place in about .8 second in most persons. The blood in the right side of the heart, shown in black has a heavy concentration of Carbon Dioxide, having come from all parts of the body. The blood in the left side of the heart is oxygenated, having come from the lungs.

A. The ventricles are empty, the blood having just left them, and the auricles are filling with blood, the auriculoventricular valves being closed.

Right side—Tricuspid valves.
Left side—Mitral valves.
A.V. side—Auricle valves.

B. The auriculoventricular valves are open and permit the blood to flow into the ventricles. At this time the blood cannot leave the ventricles because the semilunar valves in the arteries leading from them are closed.

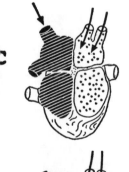

C. The ventricles are filled with blood, and the auriculoventricular valves are closed.

D. The blood is forcibly expelled from the ventricles by the contraction of their walls.

Tri.

Mit.

Mit.

A.V.

A.V.

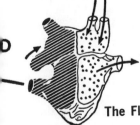

The Flow of Blood Through The Heart

Everyday the average heart, your best friend, beats 100,000 times and pumps about 2,000 gallons of blood for nourshing your body. In 70 years that adds up to more than 2.5 billion (faithful) heartbeats. Please be good to your heart and start this life–saving heart program for living a longer, healthier life!
– Patricia Bragg

"greater," goes to tissues, limbs, internal organs, and back to the heart. The other, the "lesser," goes only through the lungs and then back to the heart.

Pressure in the arteries is naturally much greater than in the veins, as it is the arteries which directly take the rush of blood when it is pumped out of the heart.

THE RHYTHMIC BEAT OF THE HEART

Because the lower part of the heart is situated slightly to the left, it is easier to hear heartbeats by listening on the left side of the chest. Actually, however, the heartbeat originates in the middle of the neck region and descends to the mid-line into the chest. The heart is in the center.

The heart-on-the-left myth is very ancient—and no matter how often refuted the legend persists. "Our ears tell us!" But they tell wrongly. The old wives' tale that it is bad to sleep on the left side for fear of compressing the heart is manifest nonsense.

A healthy heart keeps a steady rhythm in its pumping, called the *pulse*. The pulse rate is usually measured at the wrist, where one of the main arteries is near the surface. *The normal rate in an adult human being is about 72 beats per minute.* Between each beat of the heart there is 1/6 of a second rest. When a person has lived for fifty years, his heart has therefore rested eight years out of those fifty!

To keep our heart fit means that we are going to have good circulation within the blood vessels or pipes of our body and that every part of the body is going to be evenly supplied with blood. This means no cold hands or cold feet. It means that we will not suffer from every little change in the weather. It means that our body, from head to toe, will be well supplied with blood.

Walking and all forms of exercise accelerate the circulation and help prevent blockage of the blood vessels, especially the arteries. Eating more unsaturated (liquid) fats such as vegetable oils instead of saturated (hard) animal fats also helps to prevent clogging the arteries with fatty cholesterol, which will be discussed in detail later in this book.

16

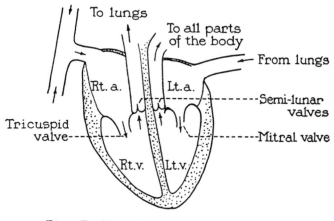

Rt.a. = Right auricle
Lt.a. = Left   "
Rt.v. = Right ventricle
Lt.v. = Left   "

Diagrammatic representation of the principal structures of the heart.

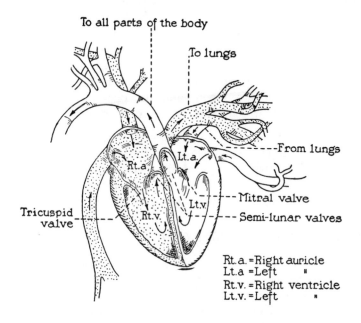

Rt.a. = Right auricle
Lt.a = Left   "
Rt.v. = Right ventricle
Lt.v. = Left   "

Longitudinal section of the heart, showing the relationship to blood vessels.

WHAT IS A HEART ATTACK?

When healthy, the human heart is a model of efficiency and perfection. But when people do not watch their diet and do not exercise every day, the walls of the arteries become cluttered with deposits of a wax-like fatty substance called cholesterol. This damages the walls of the arteries, forms scar tissue, traps more cholesterol and also mineral deposits. This condition is known as atherosclerosis.

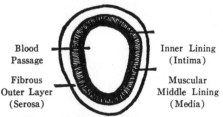

Blood Passage

Fibrous Outer Layer (Serosa)

Inner Lining (Intima)

Muscular Middle Lining (Media)

A healthy artery with a normal passage for the flow of blood.

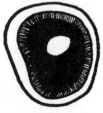

An artery showing a considerable amount of cholestrol deposits; note the narrowed passage.

Instead of being flexible and elastic as they need to be for the pulsing flow of the blood, the walls of the arteries become hard and brittle. The accumulating deposits narrow the channel through which the blood must pass. All of this slows down the circulation of the blood, and in time may cause the formation of a clot which blocks the circulation completely.

When the *clot forms in one of the arteries of the heart,* it creates a condition called coronary thrombosis or coronary occlusion. The affected part of the heart is deprived of its blood circulation. Failing to get nourishment and oxygen, it ceases to function. This is known as a heart attack.

BE PREPARED FOR EMERGENCIES

Heart attacks come suddenly. You should always be prepared for such an emergency . . . whether it happens to you or someone near you. *If you have been warned that you are a potential heart attack victim* . . . by your physician or by such symptoms as shortness of breath, chest pains, etc. . . . you should always have with you a portable oxygen supply carrier, such as "Lifogen". It is lightweight -

weighs about 3 pounds, and contains a 15-minute supply of oxygen which is easily applied, and costs around $30. . . an investment that may save your life or your love one.

If you have a healthy heart, you should be prepared to aid a heart attack victim in an emergency . . . not only to summon the paramedics or fire department or a life-guard if one is near . . . but also to give immediate emergency treatment until professional aid arrives. The Red Cross, fire departments and most high schools offer free public courses in mouth-to-mouth resuscitation and other vital first aid emergency methods. This life saving course should be a must for such knowledge may help you to save more than one human life, including someone dear to you.

WHAT IS ANGINA PECTORIS?

When one of the arteries of the heart is temporarily deprived of oxygen, it goes into a spasm. This condition is known as angina pectoris. It causes a sharp pain in the chest.

It is fortunate that these spasms last only a short time—usually no longer than a few seconds, sometimes 3 to 5 minutes, rarely more than 15 to 20 minutes.

However, if the spasm lasts for more than half a hour it is serious, and a coronary occlusion or coronary thrombosis must be suspected.

Hygiene of the excretory system

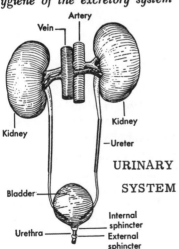

ROLE OF THE KIDNEYS IN HEART ATTACK

When the circulation into the kidneys becomes affected, their functions become seriously impaired. They are unable to eliminate the poisonous toxins efficiently, and *the fluid balance of the body becomes upset*. This in turn overtaxes the arteries of the heart, and leads to their breakdown.

19

WHAT IS A STROKE?

When a *blood clot blocks the circulation to a part of the brain,* a condition develops known as apoplexy or a "stroke." The affected part of the brain fails to receive its oxygen-enriched blood, and the part of the body which is controlled by this part of the brain becomes paralyzed.

So, you can plainly see that the statement, "A man is as old as his arteries," is quite true and not to be ignored.

WHAT CAN YOU DO—TODAY— TO REDUCE VULNERABILITY TO HEART ATTACK?

Every day in the United States there are more than *10,000 heart attacks!* You could be next—unless you are going to do something about it TODAY!

And you can start this very day to prevent a heart attack.

Now, I am the first to admit that the prevention of heart attack is basically a lifetime job of avoiding the slow deposits that clog the arteries. But if you are really serious about avoiding a heart attack there is a *Heart Fitness Program* you can start right now.

The very first thing I want you to work for are *clean arteries.* The inner lining of the healthy person's arteries is smooth and flexible so that the blood can flow through them easily.

THE IMPORTANCE OF KEEPING THE BLOOD-CHOLESTEROL LEVEL LOW

Every nation that lives on a civilized commercial diet is eating its way into the danger zone of heart attacks. Evidence from the greatest medical authorities around the world supports the shocking dangers of high blood-cholesterol levels.

The *United States* has the highest known average blood-cholesterol level in the world. And the United States is generally credited with the dubious honor of being the *birthplace of the coronary epidemic.* As things stand today, one out of every two men in the United States will die long before his time with a heart attack.

20

WORLD DEATH RATES FOR HEART DISEASE

COUNTRY	RATE	Per Cent of Fat in Relation to Total Calories	Saturated Types of Fat in Relation to Total Calories
United States	704	39.2	33.5
Finland	621	31.1	28.4
Canada	588	38.0	35.0
Australia	577	37.9	34.7
New Zealand	525	39.8	37.6
United Kingdom	428	38.4	35.0
West Germany	314	35.6	23.0
Denmark	295	38.3	25.5
Sweden	295	39.4	28.3
Austria	294	31.3	23.9
Switzerland	273	33.6	23.6
Chile	267	19.8	12.0
Belgium	250	35.0	24.4
Norway	249	38.0	17.0
Italy	226	22.3	10.5
Japan	122	7.9	1.4
France	109	29.5	20.7
Portugal	108	24.5	9.4
Ceylon	103	15.2	11.8
Yugoslavia	68	19.1	13.2

This chart illustrates the striking difference between the United States and Yugoslavia, the death rate varying by more than ten times, that is, more than 1000 per cent. The lowest six countries all use very little saturated fat, except for France (although a large number of the French use olive oil and other unsaturated fats).

AMERICANS LOVE HIGH CHOLESTEROL FOODS

American men love their big steaks, big slices of roast beef, thick slices of ham, pork chops, pork ribs, pork roasts, bacon and lunch meats ... as well as cheeses, ice cream, whipped cream, cream, milk, butter, eggs, sour cream, commercial pies and pastries, candy, fried potatoes, meat gravies, meat soups potato chips ... and all the various commercial salad dressings made from saturated oils.

21

All these favorite foods of the American diet have a preponderance of *hard or saturated fats* primarily of animal origin. These saturated fats are *high in cholesterol content,* and therefore help to raise the blood-cholesterol level. The average blood-cholesterol index in the United States today stands somewhere betwen 230 and 260—far above the "safety level." And high blood-cholesterol levels have definitely been established as the *forerunners* of the great number of heart attacks.

WHAT IS NORMAL BLOOD-CHOLESTEROL?

It is perfectly normal to have a certain amount of fat and cholesterol in the bloodstream, as these are necessary for the upkeep of the human body. It is an excess that is the trouble-maker. That is why we should keep our blood-cholesterol level normal.

How can we determine the true index of a normal blood-cholesterol level? It can to a great extent be gauged by a comparison with other peoples of the world—whole populations completely free of coronary disease. Since the onset of the "coronary epidemic" in the United States, medical experts have made exhaustive studies on this subject.

MEDICAL EXPERTS STATE "120 TO 200"

Although they differ in the range of safety in the blood-cholesterol index, top medical scientists and researchers agree in placing it at a level below 200. Here are some of the opinions:

"150 to 185" according to Dr. W. D. Wright of the University of Nebraska, College of Medicine.

"Below 200" said Dr. N. Joliffe of New York City's Department of Health.

"170" was the opinion of Dr. A. G. Shaper of the Makerere College Medical School in Uganda.

"180 as a maximum" stated Dr. Bernard Amsterdam in the New York State Journal of Medicine.

"200 or less" was the verdict of Dr. M. E. Groover in the Journal of the College of Physicians.

"150" according to Dr. Louis H. Nahum of the Yale School of Medicine.

"120 to 180" is the optimal normal, in the judgment of Dr. William Dock, Professor of Medicine at the State University of New York.

In my opinion, I believe that the blood-cholesterol level of "120 to 180" as given by Dr. Dock is about correct. In my own personal life this is the level at which I keep my blood-cholesterol.

It is my suggestion that you *get your blood-cholesterol test at least once a year*. Twice is better ... for it is better to be safe than to be sorry.

FASTING IS THE QUICKEST WAY
TO LOWER BLOOD-CHOLESTEROL NATURALLY

In my opinion, fasting is the quickest and the easiest method of lowering blood-cholesterol. I get my test for blood-cholesterol twice a year, and if it goes over 180 I fast from 3 to 7 days and it soon goes back below 180.

Fasting is a wonderful way to give the heart a rest. That is why I fast for a 24-hour period every week on distilled water. I will discuss this in more detail later in this book.

(NOTE: For full and complete details on the Science of Fasting, read my book *THE MIRACLE OF FASTING*. See inside back cover of this book for information on obtaining it.)

The elimination of waste products by Fasting increases longevity.
Alexis Carrel, M.D., Famous Scientist

CHOLESTEROL—THE BAROMETER OF OUR LIFESPAN

The one thing that will unquestionably shorten the life span is a body that is overburdened with blood fat, or what is known as an excess of cholesterol.

Cholesterol in itself is not harmful. In fact, it is important to many of our body processes, and the body even manufactures it as extra fuel in emergencies. "Chole" means bile, and "sterol" means fatty. Much of the fat that we eat is broken down by the liver into cholesterol and excreted into the bile, later to be reabsorbed into the bloodstream for distribution to the tissues. As noted, normal blood-cholesterol levels are 120 to 180.

But when our diet is *overloaded* with the high cholesterol content of saturated (hard) animal fats, and when we do not exercise enough to burn up even the normal—much less the excess—amount of cholesterol as fuel . . . then *the bloodstream becomes "choked"* with the waxy particles of cholesterol, which lodge in the arterial walls and clog them. It has been established that the amount of cholesterol deposited in the walls of the arteries is in direct relationship to the amount of cholesterol in the bloodstream.

Thus you can see how clogged the arteries must be when the blood-cholesterol level rises to 270, 320, 380 and even higher! Yet these excessive levels are not uncommon today, especially in American men.

Remember that the amount of cholesterol in your blood tells you of the risk you are running of having a coronary ailment or attack. It is *the barometer of your life-span.*

It is very wise, therefore, for every adult to see to it that he does not raise his blood-cholesterol above a safe normal level. These chunks of waxy cholesterol can block an artery and bring on heart failure, stroke or even death!

HOW MUCH FATS ARE YOU STOWING AWAY?

Most persons know little or nothing about cholesterol, and go merrily on using large quantities of butter on their bread, toast, buns, potatoes and vegetables. They drink great quantities of pasteurized milk and gobble gallons of ice cream.

24

Meat, fish, poultry, egg yolks, potato chips, French fried potatoes, doughnuts, bacon, ham and sausage pour fat into the blood. Little do people realize that their high levels of cholesterol are leading them to disaster ... that they *may be literally "eating themselves to death."*

Some individuals consume as many as 4 or 5 cups of saturated fats daily ... and then wonder why they have a heart attack, a stroke or some other form of heart trouble!

As I mentioned previously, the clogging of the arterial system by excess cholesterol—the deposits of heavy, waxy fat in the walls of the arteries—is called *atherosclerosis. It is not brought on by age, but by diet!* Examination of the bodies of young soldiers killed in battle in Korea revealed the shocking fact that 77% of the Americans (average age 22) already had atherosclerosis. In contrast, among the Koreans and other Orientals who had died on the same battlefield under the same conditions, there was only 11% incidence of this disease. As is well known, the Oriental diet is low in saturated fats.

THE DEADLY FATS

The United States is a nation of fat-eaters. 40% of the average American diet is made up of *saturated* fats—and most of these are *commercial hydrogenated fats,* the *most deadly* of all fats!

Commercial hydrogenated fat is not a natural fat in any sense of the word. It is a solid fat—so solid that it cannot be broken down by the body heat, which is 98.6 degrees.

Natural, unsaturated fats break down at body temperature. These are actually perishable food. In time, natural unsaturated fats will take on oxygen and become rancid, with a strong odor and bitter taste which makes them unappetizing for human consumption.

Hydrogenated, saturated fat remains "stable" because it has been made impervious to oxygen. In reality, it is embalmed fat. Yet the American housewife has been brainwashed by the large manufacturers of these saturated, hydrogenated fats into believing that they are permanently "fresh!"

25

She can buy a can of one of the well known brands and keep it in the house from one to ten years, because it is impossible for it to turn rancid. Clever advertising tells her that these saturated, hydrogenated, snow white, heavily processed vegetable shortenings will not smoke . . . and there is other sales prattle which has no relation whatsoever to good nutrition. The same applies to margarine made to imitate butter.

So—instead of the natural, unsaturated fats that will aid her family's health—she feeds her loved ones these deadly saturated, hydrogenated fats that are nothing but trouble makers when an excess gets into the bloodstream. High in cholesterol content, these "killer" fats clog up the human pipe system, especially the vital arteries, and can eventually cause a fatal or crippling clot (thrombosis).

Beware of saturated, hydrogenated fats!

LISTEN TO THE WORDS OF DR. PAUL DUDLEY WHITE— THE GREAT HEART SPECIALIST

Dr. Paul Dudley White, past president of the American Heart Association and world famous heart specialist, has wise advice to give on taking care of the heart. I want to call your attention especially to the following points made by Dr. White in an article written for the Heart Association. He begins with the startling information that *middle age begins at 20* and the *"dangerous years"* are ages 20 to 40. Here are Dr. White's own words:

"When does middle age begin? At 20, and it lasts until 80. And the dangerous years of this 60-year span are the *first 20*, not the last. *These are the years when an overfed and under-exercised public is sowing the seeds of a coronary harvest.*"

UNLIMITED LIFE EXPECTANCY POSSIBLE— SAYS DR. WHITE

"I conceive the ages of man as five," Dr. White continues. "Birth to the 20th year; then a three-stage middle age of 20 to 40, 40 to 60, and 60 to 80; and finally old age—80 to 100. The latter constitutes a steadily expanding horizon to which I see no eventual limit. *Our life expectancy should keep rising*

26

indefinitely as scientific research keeps making progress against disease.

"The public can play an important role in this effort to push the life-span farther and farther. *Individual physical-fitness and nutritional programs for men and women between the ages of 24 and 40 would guard against creeping degeneration and would instill lifelong good health habits* . . .

"A man marries in his early 20's; his wife cooks too much and too well—and between her cooking, the family car and the TV set, the man has gained 20 pounds—or maybe 30—by the time he's 45. These are the years in which atherosclerosis (cholesterol blocking and clogging the arteries) and rusting of the arteries occur—and it can ultimately reach the brain as a stroke, or the heart as a coronary thrombosis (massive blood clot). It may affect the kidneys. This is why an apparently healthy man drops dead at 45 or 50. *His death is not sudden at all; it's been building up for years* . . .

"The automobile and the TV, I might add, should be the servants of the American public, not its masters . . .

"Despite the nation's generally unhealthy way of life, two factors work in favor of the American person in his forties," Dr. White concludes. *"It is never too late—at any age—to begin controlling obesity and resuming a program of sensible exercise* . . . One excellent form, available to all, is walking. This should be brisk, and for a normally healthy person five miles is not enough. Neither is one weekly 18-hole golf game."

(NOTE: Dr. White is a great bicycle enthusiast and even in his 80's he pedals miles at a time.)

There you have it—from a world famous heart specialist. *Exercise and diet.* Both should—and can—be regular and enjoyable, as you will discover by following the Heart Fitness Program outlined in this book.

DR. CARREL'S AMAZING DISCOVERY

The eminent biologist, *Dr. Alexis Carrel* of the Rockefeller Research Institute in New York City, *proved* to the world that *living flesh can be deathless!*

In January 1912 this great scientist took a sliver of a heart muscle from an embryo chicken and provided it with two essentials—simple protein food and correct drainage of the tissue. In this laboratory experiment, this tiny bit of embryo heart flesh was kept alive for more than 35 years ... and it lasted long enough to prove that it could be continued indefinitely. When the experiment was terminated in 1947, this fragment of heart tissue had lived many lifetimes of a chicken—the equivalent, in fact, of hundreds of years of human life. It was called the "tissue of eternal youth."

This amazing bit of embryo heart flesh doubled its size every 48 hours! Slices had to be cut away and discarded every day, because the continuing growth to a huge size would make it impossible to feed and cleanse the living heart cells. For more than 35 years at the Rockefeller Institute any scientific man could observe "eternal life" before his very eyes!

We can learn a great lessson from Dr. Carrel's outstanding scientific demonstration of the chicken heart—namely, that *if the body is correctly fed and drainage is provided for the poisons, life can go on indefinitely.*

IT'S UP TO YOU!

You—and only you—can take the proper care of your heart and your body, so that you may enjoy the "prime of your life" indefinitely. Most people reach their "prime" between 25 and 35, and then there is a sharp decline.

I maintain that any person who will follow this Heart Fitness Program can attain the prime of life at any age—and maintain that prime for many years.

If you have high blood pressure or low blood pressure, you can restore it to normal by following the Natural Laws that keep your heart in good condition. My own blood pressure is 120 systolic over 80 diastolic——the same level as that of a perfectly healthy young man in his 20's. My pulse rate is in the 60's and steady.

I know that my case is not an isolated one—I am not a freak. In my many years in Nutrition and Physical Culture I have met many men and women in almost unbelievably good physical condition at great calendar ages.

28

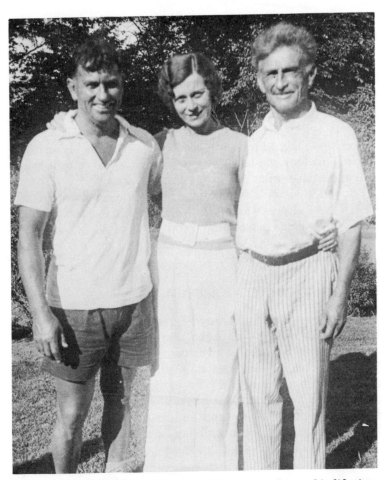

Paul C. Bragg (left) at the turn of the century began his life-time career in Natural Physical Fitness with the famous Physical Culture pioneer, Bernarr Macfadden (right). Bragg was editor of Macfadden's Physical Culture Magazine, which was the first publication to bring the basic principles of healthful living to popular attention in the U.S.A. He is credited with "getting women out of bloomers into shorts, and men into bathing trunks." Bragg was also active with Macfadden's "Penny Kitchen Restaurants" during the Depression era, when they fed millions of hungry people. Bragg helped develop America's first Health Spa at Dansville, New York, where the above photo was taken, and then opened in Florida, Macfadden's Deauville Hotel which gave undeveloped Miami Beach its great beginning. Macfadden was the father of Physical Culture in America, and Bragg the father of the Health Movement and originator of Health Food Stores.

MACFADDEN—FOUNDER OF PHYSICAL CULTURE

At one time I was associated with Bernarr Macfadden, "father" and founder of the Physical Culture Movement. Mr. Macfadden spent thousands of dollars in an attempt to find the *oldest living humans* on the face of the earth.

I was selected as his researcher on this project. Every person who claimed an advanced age was thoroughly investigated. This took me to many parts of the world, interviewing men and women from *110 to 154 years of age!*

I found this work fascinating, because deep down in my heart I have always wanted to live a long life . . . not the long life of the average person which ends at 70 or 80 . . . but a life that would last 130, 140 or 150 years. And my research has proved that it can be done!

ZORA AGHA—ACTIVE AT AGE 154

In Constantinople, Turkey, I met and talked with an amazing man named Zora Agha who was 154 years old. And what was this remarkable man doing at age 154? He was a baggage porter for the large railroad station in Constantinople! For 12 hours every day he carried heavy baggage! His eyesight, his hearing and his physical strength were unbelievable. His mind was keen and he had a sense of humor that kept him joking and smiling all day long.

In the 154 years of his life he had lost only two teeth. When he showed me his teeth and gums I was amazed. Every tooth in his head looked like a pearl . . . strong, white and hard.

ZORA AGHA'S SECRET OF YOUTH— NATURAL FOOD AND EXERCISE

Through an interpreter I questioned Zora Agha about the secrets of his astounding long and healthy life. *His whole diet was simple* and not complicated by the use of any refined or processed foods. He had never in his life eaten refined white bread or refined white sugar and, being a Moslem, he had never tasted alcoholic drinks of any kind.

When I asked him what was his favorite food, he replied readily, "*Dates.*" This had been verified by some of my other research on long-lived, healthy people. I have discovered that people who eat dates have an abundance of vital energy, stamina and endurance. At one time in the Atlas Mountains of North Africa, I investigated a tribe of primitive Arabs who astonished me with their extraordinary strength. I met men 70, 80 and 90 years of age who were expert horsemen and could spend days in the African heat of 120° to 130°.

But it was from Zora Agha in faroff Turkey that I first learned the amazing value of dates as a healthful food. I also learned that he limited himself to 3 or 4 dates at a time. He knew the remarkable energy value of the *natural sugars found in dates*, but he also knew that the body has only a limited capacity for handling these sugars.

ZORA'S DIET LIKE THAT OF BIBLICAL TIMES

The vigorous 154-year-old Zora Agha also ate a large amount of *garlic*, one of the "forgotten foods" of man. Garlic has been called *"the poor man's penicillin"* . . . and as a Nutritionist, I know its value in helping to keep the heart and arteries fit.

Zora told me that he ate only stale *black bread that had been dried in the sunshine.* He would purchase a loaf of black bread, slice it and let it dry in the sun. He never ate fresh bread. (NOTE: When we are traveling, my daughter, Patricia, dries our health bread in the sunshine by simply putting it out on the window sill. So, even when you are away from home, you can eat healthy, dried bread.)

Other items of Zora Agha's diet included *lean meat, ripe olives* and plenty of *fruits* and *vegetables.* He did not use butter and never ate more than two eggs weekly. The only oil he used for cooking and on his salads was *safflower oil.* This oil has been used in Turkey and throughout Asia Minor, as well as in the Holy Land, for hundreds of years.

Zora's only beverage besides *water* was *mint tea*, which is the national beverage of all Arabs and Moslems.

It seemed to me that Zora Agha had naturally discovered the secret of longevity of the old Biblical patriarchs who lived to such fabulous ages, and whose diet was so much like his.

LIFE DEPENDS UPON THE FOOD WE EAT

From this 154-year-old, healthy, energetic man I learned a great deal about keeping the heart fit—by a simple diet of natural foods, lean meats and plenty of vigorous exercise.

I have met only one Zora Agha in my lifetime ... but I know that when the mass of civilized mankind adopts simple, natural diets there will be vast numbers of people who will reach his remarkable age of 154 years.

Every intelligent person will agree that life depends largely upon the food we eat. How sound and well selected our foods are may logically foreshadow how sound our heart, body cells, brain, tissues and vital organs will be tomorrow, next mouth, next year, and ten years from now. *The chemistry of the food a person eats becomes his own body chemistry.* This includes the chemistry of the heart, brain, nerves and the entire body.

BLOOD—THE RIVER OF LIFE

The body is composed of billions of tiny cells that are nourished by the blood from the food we eat. As we read in the Bible: *"The life of the flesh is in the blood." (Lev. 17:11)* If we can keep the vital eight quarts of blood in our body in perfect chemical balance—so that our vital organs and all the cells of our tissues are properly nourished—and if we keep the pipes of the body free from corrosion, there is no reason why we cannot have many, many years of "youthful" living. Good blood and good circulation are the answer to a long life free from premature debility.

You can start today to follow this philosophy by realizing that *all the red blood cells* in the bloodstream undergo a *complete change every 28 days.* They renew themselves through a series of births (and deaths) about 12 times a year ... and this process continues from the cradle to the grave.

Our red blood cells are manufactured chiefly from the food we eat and the beverages we drink. Is it not logical that if we put the correct nutriments into our bodies and keep the "pipes" (arteries, veins, capillaries) clean and free from corrosion, we can increase our life span?

32

YOU CAN CONTROL YOUR OWN
BIOLOGIC "CLOCK OF LIFE"

You cannot get sound health from any other source than from healthy, circulating blood nourished by correct food, air and liquids. These substances must be actively distributed throughout your body by the heart and blood vessels.

It is my contention that any person—regardless of age or physical condition —can rebuild himself and have a strong heart and clean "pipes." I have demonstrated this in my own body. My own abundant health, strength, endurance and stamina are the best proofs of the success I have had in rebuilding my body from a hopeless, helpless physical wreck into sound super-health, efficient cardiac function and vigorous arterial and venal circulation.

Do not be discouraged by your physical condition. Remember that *the body is self-repairing, self-healing, and self-maintaining.* "Where there's life, there's hope" . . . and by working with Mother Nature you can rebuild a new bloodstream ... and with a new bloodstream you can build a fit heart. To live long you must have a strong heart and you must have blood vessels that are flexible, elastic and clean. *This Heart Fitness Program is your blueprint to a new YOU!* —vital, fresh, sparkling!

Age is not a matter of how many years you have lived. It resolves itself into how clean your arteries are and the chemical condition of your blood. *You can control your own biologic "clock of life"* . . . and there is no reason why you cannot fulfill the Biblical prophecy:

"Man's days shall be 120 years." (Genesis 6:3).

"OLD AGE" IS NOT NECESSARY

Why grow old? "Old age" is not necessary—at least not so necessary as you may think. Instead of submissively "growing old" . . . *revolt! Grow young!* You can defy time, "steal a march" on it. At 60 you can be bright-eyed as a bird and radiate the joy of living ... at 70 you can be supple and full of sunny cheer ... at 80 you can wear age like a jewel ... and who knows, you may become a second Zora Agha!

It's up to you. You stand at life's crossroads. Will you take the line of least resistance that can lead only to a premature end ... or will you, by disciplined living, climb to the clear heights of a healthful life? If you are going to strive for longevity, begin today ... BEGIN RIGHT NOW!

YOU CAN GROW YOUNG—IF YOU WANT TO

Why not "grow young"? If you have the wish and the desire, you have the power ... and by the Great Goddess of Health, Hygeia, you will succeed!

In this Heart Fitness Program *I am going to help you* to have a powerful heart, a chemically balanced bloodstream and a strong circulatory system. *I cannot do it for you.* I have no "specifics," no "cures" for a diseased heart. *Only Nature has the power* to heal a diseased heart. But if we will give our bloodstream the proper building materials, we can build a fit body.

Regard this Heart Fitness Program as one of inspiration. It is to induce you to take stock, get a fresh grip and hoist yourself onto a higher plane of Health and Happiness.

THE HIGHWAY TO HIGH HEALTH

Health and Happiness! ... To me these seem inseparable. My motto is:

"To make my body a temple pure wherein I live serene."

With me the welfare of my heart and my body is a religion. But by Health I do not mean the everyday variety that consists in "not being actually sick." I mean what I call "High Health" . . . the sense of superlative wellbeing that makes a person slap himself on the chest and say with gusto, "I am feeling fine today!"

We all agree that the chief aim of life is happiness. There is but one avenue to happiness which can be recommended with reasonable confidence ... and that is the Highway to High Health! *Without health there can be no constant happiness.*

One can think of happiness as arising from health alone. The lusty ditchdigger is more in love with life than the flabby, sick millionaire. Good Health is the prime factor in attaining Happiness. Keep your body fit and your mind will rejoice.

34

A HEALTHY BODY AND A HAPPY MIND

A happy, healthy body usually means a happy, healthy mind. It by no means follows, however, that a happy mind will make a happy body. It would be glorious if the spirit could so triumph over the flesh. But alas! ... the condition of the body usually has greater influence upon the mind than the mind has upon the body. A person with a perfectly sound body will seldom be miserable ... but it is rare for a sick person to be conspicuously gay.

Men and women today are slowing down the aging proces by living healthier lives. Life expectancy today is up to 120 years. The human structure is mechanically adapted for full energies and activities at 70 and 80, clearly proven by the increase of men and women nationwide who are hale, hearty, springy of step, clear of eye and keen of mind who live well into their golden years. If we want to get the maximum fun out of life, let us begin with this body of ours.

That is why I am, first and foremost, a Nutritional and Physical Culture enthusiast. Happiness is largely dependent upon the care we give our bodies. *Through the harmony of the flesh we achieve the exultation of the spirit. Mental serenity is profoundly physical in its source* ... and by the purification of the living tissue we are helped to attain the Higher Life.

Let us therefore put the health of our body and heart before everything, as everything else depends upon this.

IT IS NEVER TOO LATE TO LEARN

Would you trust the repair of your car to someone who had no knowledge of mechanics? Of course not! Yet in regard to the precious mechanism of the human body, that is exactly what the average person is doing.

Fortunately, *it is never too late to obtain and apply knowledge*. I have already described to you the structure and functioning of the human heart and circulatory system (pages 10-17) and explained the importance of keeping the blood-cholesterol at a normally low level (pages 20-25). I suggest that you review these pages from time to time, so that you will thoroughly understand the *why* of the Heart Fitness Program which I am going to outline for you. Let this Program be your guide on the Highway to High Health.

35

THE DISCOVERY OF HEALTH

Health has been defined as "physical unconsciousness" . . . and although all physical unconsciousness is not health, the greatest compliment we can pay to the functioning of our body is to be unaware of it because it is running so smoothly. Most young people do not realize there is such a thing as health because they have it in abundance.

With the years, however, we tend to become more and more "health-conscious." This adage is so often true: "You spend your Health to gain your Wealth" . . . and in later life, its reverse: "You spend your Wealth to regain your Health." The health-conscious person usually becomes so after being sick . . . and I am of the opinion that most people over 50 are a little sick. There would be no such thing as health if it were not for the lack of it . . . and we begin to discover its existence just when we need it most.

But while "health consciousness" may often be due to impaired vitality, let me suggest that this applies only to the common variety of health. High Health is essentially conscious . . . or rather, it is "conscious of its unconsciousness." It is *health-pride—something to be cherished*. It is a manifestation of the will and deep desire to live a long, happy and healthfully active life.

FOR SECURITY AND HAPPINESS—
INVEST IN THE "BANK OF HEALTH"

Can you think of any greater comfort, security and happiness that could come to you than the confident belief that you need never be ill? Or that your loved ones need never be stricken with heart disease? That no one need die at an early age, unless by accident?

Perhaps this seems "too good to be true" . . . yet this ideal state of affairs is possible of attainment by anyone willing to apply the principles of this Heart Fitness Program. It is my sincere conviction, and I say it to you in all seriousness, that the tragically prevalent heart diseases, as well as many other diseases, are entirely unnecessary and are strictly within one's own control to prevent if we only make the effort.

36

Let health become a definite study with you. The time and effort you spend in following this Heart Fitness Program will be an investment in the "Bank of Health" that can bring you and your loved ones great happiness and security. Health is Wealth!

The teachings contained in this Program—if followed faithfully and conscientiously—cannot fail to result in acquiring and maintaining a youthful feeling and a fit heart.

Again let me emphasize that this Heart Fitness Program is not a cure for heart disease . . . nor can this Program do anything until it is applied. But the body can heal itself if given a chance, as has been proved in thousands of cases.

THE BIG THREE FOR A HEALTHY HEART AND LONG LIFE— 1) NORMAL WEIGHT 2) DAILY EXERCISE 3) PROPER DIET

Suppose you were told that you had to lug an unwieldy load of 20-to-50 pounds around with you wherever you went— walking, sitting, eating, sleeping—all day and all night. How would you feel about it? You would protest indignantly, wouldn't you?

Yet that is exactly what you are doing when you are overweight! You are carrying around a load of unhealthy, flabby blubber. You are overtaxing all the functions of your body—especially your heart and circulatory system.

Excess fat is dangerous! It exhausts the heart. Insurance statistics show that fat people are the shortest lived. Every pound of excess fat on your body shortens your life. That is why *the No. 1 Rule for a Healthy Heart is Normal Weight.*

This normal weight must be naturally attained and maintained. Drugs can be even more dangerous than fat!

Rule No. 2 for a Healthy Heart is Daily Exercise. The proper exercise will not only help you to keep your weight naturally normal. It will also stimulate healthful circulation of the blood throughout your body . . . tone up your muscles and vital organs . . . aid all the functions of your body . . . and help bring you the glow of radiant Health.

If the next pasture looks greener it may be because it's getting better care.

Most important of all is Rule No. 3—Proper Diet! A healthy heart and a healthy body depend upon clean, healthy blood ... and clean, healthy blood depends upon the food you eat. I will discuss all of these points in detail, and in listing Proper Diet as No. 3 I am "saving the best for last." Your diet is the most important factor in controlling your weight ... nourishing your blood and through it the rest of your body ... protecting your heart from deadly cholesterol and strengthening it to become a powerful "fountain of life" and "fountain of eternal youth."

BEWARE OF EXCESS FAT

A normal amount of fatty tissue is an indication of health. But when fatty accumulations begin to bulge out here and there and destroy youthful outlines—beware! These are danger signals warning you that it is time to take action.

Overweight invites heart attacks. It puts an undue strain upon your heart ... and it also indicates that you have been eating saturated fats that clog your arteries with cholesterol.

Excess fat is fatal to beauty. Excess fat is fatal to youth. Excess fat brings on disease or premature death.

The old myth that full red cheeks and a plump or fat body are indications of health still persists, even in this enlightened age. The myth dies hard—but the fat person dies easily. Disease gains a foothold more readily and is more difficult to dislodge.

Fat people are inclined to be slow and phlegmatic. The excess fat on the body indicates similar accumulations around the heart, kidneys and other vital organs, impairing their function. *Life itself depends upon the functional processes performed by the heart and vital organs. If their activities are hindered by excess fat the body suffers throughout its every part.*

Our ancestors are wished on us, but our habits, good or bad, are something we can control. —Edward J. Stieglitz, M.D.

DON'T BE A "FAT-HEAD"

To be called a "fat-head" is an unpardonable insult. It reflects upon your intelligence. But what could be more un-intelligent than allowing your body to be encumbered by ugly, unhealthy, dangerous blubber? Surely the time will come when "fat-bodied" and "fat-head" will become synonymous and considered equally disgraceful!

A fat person is sluggish and slow. His vital resistance is usually low. If speed is necessary, he puffs like a steam engine. His heart and lungs are inefficient, not equal to emergencies. A fat person moves about with difficulty, and his load of surplus weight lessens his mental as well as his physical activity.

When an athlete is training for a contest, he eliminates from his body all extra fat. He understands that it is in his way and will lessen his endurance and decrease his physical energies. In the military services the same applies.

A fat man cannot fight well—and in every sphere of endeavor a fighter is needed. Inefficiency and fat are cronies . . . they sleep together and eat together . . . but they do not exercise together!

YOUR WAISTLINE IS YOUR LIFELINE
AND YOUR DATELINE

When you are fat you are flirting with old age. You are allowing the old age cells to gather in your body. You are playing with disease, and you should be prepared to pay the penalty.

Youthful bodily outlines must be maintained . . . and this requires proper care of the human machine. The rewards are well worth the effort! If you find fatty tissue accumulating, you should either increase your exercise or reduce the quantity of food you are eating—or both! Don't settle down with the satisfied feeling that fatty surplus must be expected with advancing years! If you make this mistake, old age will come much faster . . . and so will serious illness or possibly early death.

Fight excess fat as you would your deadliest enemy! It often comes upon you like a thief in the night, silently and without warning. Sometimes you realize your danger only when serious difficulties actually stare you in the face . . . then the fight is tougher. But fight you must! Your life may well depend upon it.

KEEP SLIM AND KEEP YOUR SELF-ESTEEM

A fat, unshapely body not only can destroy your health . . . it can also destroy your self-esteem. You need to be proud of your body, not ashamed of it.

Self-esteem is as necessary to the spirit as healthful food is to the body. If you want to be efficient, youthful, enthusiastic, full of the fire and fervor of life . . . keep slim and keep your self-esteem!

Build your body as an artist paints a picture or a sculptor molds a statue. Make it an expression of the best there is within you. Let it reflect your very soul—and then excess fat will find no lodgment.

WHAT IS NORMAL WEIGHT?

There are numerous charts, tables and statistics on the subject of normal weight for certain ages, heights, etc. These are based on averages. But *there is no such thing as an average person.* You may use such statistics as a general guide, but they should not be applied arbitrarily.

If you give your body the proper diet and the proper exercise, you will attain and maintain your own naturally normal weight. To weigh a certain number of pounds does not necessarily indicate the proper inch measurement of waist, hips, etc. If your flesh is firm and healthy, without excess fat, it does not matter whether you weigh more or less than the "average" for your years and height. What is important is to find your own natural, normal weight as the result of proper care of your body. If your body is healthy and fit, your weight is normal—for YOU. *Flabby fat is never normal!*

The saying, *"If you don't use it, you lose it,"* certainly applies to the 600 muscles of the human body. When not used, they lose their muscle tone and become fat and flabby.

MIND OVER MATTER

Make up your mind that you really want to slim down to your naturally normal weight. This is more difficult than it seems, because the mind has a way of making excuses for an overweight body. For instance, you may say to yourself, "It's normal for me to be fat. I'm the plump type." . . . or, "I eat so little, yet I remain fat." The latter may be true—but remember it is what you eat not how much. And it is never normal to be fat!

Your mind must be the boss of your body. Flesh is dumb . . . flesh is weak . . . flesh often demands fatty, starchy, sugary foods. Either your mind rules the body or the body rules the mind. Be positive! Tell your body that your mind is the absolute master.

Remember it is the lean horse for a long race. If you want a long, healthy life . . . keep your body trim and fit. Once you have trimmed down to your normal weight through proper diet and exercise, what a difference in the way you will feel! Bubbling over with vitality and energy . . . unafraid of life's challenges . . . and free from the fear of heart attack or other illness.

(NOTE: The New Bragg book on *HOW TO REDUCE— NATURE'S WAY* gives you a complete Natural Reducing Program. See inside back cover of this book for details.)

EXERCISE DAILY FOR A POWERFUL HEART

Laziness is a vicious habit. Sitting too much is a bad health habit. You need a *1 to 2-hour period every day* of your life when you can do some kind of vigorous exercise. The simplest is brisk walking, preferably up and down hills. There is no better exercise for building a strong heart than hill climbing.

I am a mountain climber. Near my home in Hollywood, California is the famous Griffith Park in which Mt. Hollywood rises some 2,000 feet. I often climb this mountain and run all the way down. At my California Desert home near Palm Springs, I am surrounded by mountains of all sizes which I enjoy climbing.

I am a walker and a jogger. Every day of my life I run and walk. I also have a bicycle which I ride for miles at a time. I swim. I play tennis. And three times a week I take my progressive weight training workout using dumbells and barbells of various weights.

Exercise is the greatest single factor available to man to remove the blockage and clogging in the arteries and other blood vessels and to increase the greater flow of oxygen-enriched blood in and through the heart and body.

DEVELOP STRENGTH FROM THE INSIDE OUT, NOT FROM THE OUTSIDE IN

Remember that from the day you were born to the day you die, your 600 muscles play an important role in everything you do ... *more than half your body is sheer muscle.*

It isn't the muscles that you see that count as much as those you don't see. Along the 30 feet of your gastro-intestinal tract there are muscles to force food along this 30-foot tube. To bring an adequate amount of air into your lungs requires strong muscles.

And above all, *the greatest muscle*—seen or unseen—in your body is *the HEART*. It is the heart that pumps the blood supply into the body's 600 muscles ... and the more we bring these 600 muscles into play, the better our heart, the better our circulation, the better our physical condition, and the better our entire state of health will be.

Without hesitation I tell you that brisk walking is the best form of exercise. You must become a prodigious pedestrian if you want to be strong from the inside out.

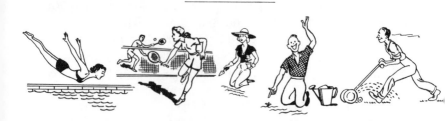

Exercise for Health

WALKING—THE "KING" OF EXERCISE

Of all forms of exercise brisk walking is the one that *brings most of the body into action.* As you walk, grasp yourself in the small of the back and feel how the entire frame responds to every stride ... how almost all your chief muscles are functioning rhythmically. In no other exercise do you get the same harmony of coordinating sinews, the same perfect circulation of the blood. Brisk walking is the "king" of exercise, ideal for you ... and your heart!

You should try to *walk 3 to 5 miles every day*, and be capable of doubling it. Don't give yourself excuses. *Make your daily walk a fixed item in your Heart Fitness Program*—all the year around and in any kind of weather. Walking requires no special equipment, and it can be done any time during your waking hours. Regardless of what other exercise you may take, your daily walk is a "must!" Walking can be done by anyone, anytime, anywhere.

Of course, you may take it in the form of golf, if you enjoy this social sport. But you must never, never ride around the golf course in an electric cart! This makes a farce of the whole thing. Walking is what your heart needs. Although I am inclined to agree with Mark Twain, who said, "Golf is a good way to spoil a good walk" ... if it takes the game to make you walk, by all means do so. The result is the same—healthily functioning muscles and quickened blood circulation with its attendant sense of harmony and happiness.

Although preferable outdoors, indoor walking is far better than none at all—in your hallway, on your porch or wherever you can get the most fresh air.

When traveling around the world on my lecture tours, I often take a late evening walk through the corridors and up and down the stairs of my hotel. If there is a roof terrace available, I prefer this.

ENJOY YOUR DAILY HIKE

Your walking should never be done selfconsciously. No heel and toe business. No getting there in a certain time. Let it be what it is—the most functional of exercises.

Walk naturally—with head high, back hollow, chest out, tummy in. Swing your hips into action and your body, too ... walk as though your legs began at the middle of your torso. Breathe deeply. You will get such a feeling of physical elation that you will carry yourself proudly—straight, erect, arms swinging easily from your shoulders.

Go your own gait, with a free spirit and a light heart. If the outer world of Nature fails to interest you, turn to the inner world of the mind. As you walk your body ceases to matter, and you become as near poet and philosopher as you will ever be. You can truly "walk your worries away." As the blood courses through your arteries and veins cleansing and nourishing your entire body, you are filled with a sense of wellbeing that cleanses your mind of its troubles and nourishes it with positive thoughts. Often as I stride along on my daily hike, I say to myself—and sometimes even aloud with each step—"Health ... Strength ... Youth ... Vitality."

It is very beneficial to take a hiking tour once a year. Select some interesting part of the country which you would like to see, and hike about 15 miles per day. In this way you will broaden your knowledge of your native land and of nature, as well as help to build a powerful, long-lasting heart.

UNCOMPLICATE YOUR LIVING

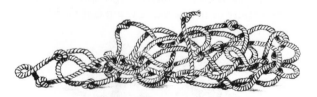

Living is a continual lesson in problem solving, but the trick is to know where to start. No excuses—start your Health Program Today.

RUN FOR YOUR LIFE

Every day I run for my life—because a *run a day may help keep heart attacks away!* This type of running is known as jogging, as practiced by many athletes in training workouts— a steady, easily sustained pace with head up, shoulders back, arms swinging naturally. Boxers, baseball players, soccer and football players—in fact, all athletes consider running or jogging as the perfect conditioner. It is standard on programs of physical training the world over.

I have been "running for my life" every day of my life for over *80* years. When I am on my world lecture tours the first question I ask the hotel manager is, "Where is the nearest park where I can take my daily jogging and running?" And off I go sometime during the day. I prefer early morning or late afternoon. Each person, however, should choose the time best suited for him.

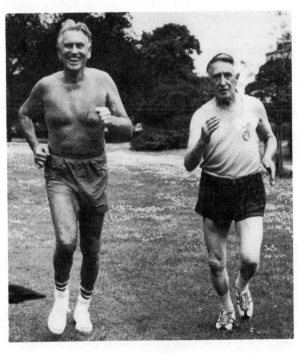

Paul C. Bragg and Duncan McLean, England's oldest Champion Sprinter (83 years young) on a training run in London's famous Regent's Park.

I have been pleased to find that all over the world today running or jogging has become an accepted method in the pursuit of Heart Fitness by persons of all age groups. Many cities have "jogging clubs" which anyone may join. I have had the pleasure of running with men and women in New Zealand, Australia and England, as well as in many parts of the United States.

In the promotion of physical, mental and emotional health, it is universally accepted that exercise is important. A daily run or jog, when adapted to the individual's physical condition and age, will improve endurance, produce a sense of wellbeing and help to maintain total body fitness. It will increase resistance to sickness and disease, help to make the heart strong and aid in prolonging life.

Before starting this type of exercise, and at all stages, it is a very wise precaution to seek the advice of a doctor, whether Medical, Chiropractor or Naturopath.

EXERCISE—THE BEST FITNESS CONDITIONER

A daily running, jogging or walking program is quick, sure and inexpensive as a fitness conditioner. You must be faithful to your Heart Fitness Program for true success.

Women will be the most pleased when they see fat weight change to lean weight, and lose inches off their waistlines and hiplines, all while improving their health.

Men and women, you both must remember your waistline is your lifeline and also your dateline! A person with a trim and fit figure always looks more youthful and attractive in his/her clothes.

If you are a "softie" and feel you cannot get outside for your run or jog on cold and rainy days—do stationary jogging (stay in one place and lift one foot at a time about 8 inches from the floor—best to start easy and buildup gradually to faster and longer periods), where you get the most fresh air— patio, front porch, hallway, or if at work, in the lounge.

A man is as old as his arteries. —Virchow

EXERCISING IN THE SKY

I even get my jogging in while I'm thousands of feet high in the air, soaring the skies in a "jet" plane. I just go to the rear of the aisle and jog. You can learn to take advantage of spare moments for stationary jogging during the day, even if you are an office worker, housewife or president of a corporation. We all must have daily exercises for heart and body fitness.

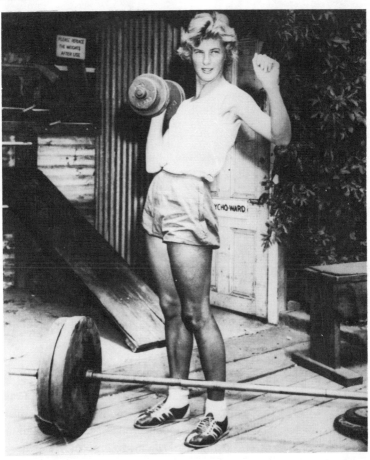

Betty Cuthbert of Sydney, Australia, "Golden Girl" of the Olympics and an enthusiastic Bragg Health Student. She has won 4 Olympic gold medals, 1 Commonwealth Games gold medal, 2 silver medals and 16 world records in almost every womens track world record from 60 metres to 440 yards.

47

WHEN YOU ARE HEALTHY AND FIT
YOU ARE HAPPY!

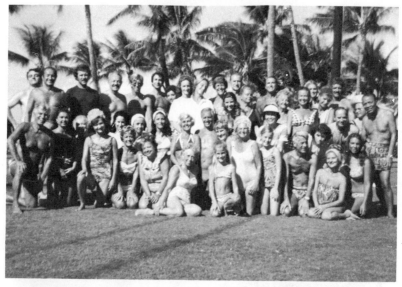

BRAGG LONGER LIFE, HEALTH AND HAPPINESS CLUB

JOIN THE FUN AT THE BRAGG "LONGER LIFE, HEALTH &
HAPPINESS CLUB" WHEN YOU VISIT HAWAII – IT'S FREE!

Paul C. Bragg, daughter Patricia and their wonderful healthy members
of the Bragg "Longer Life, Health and Happiness Club" exercise daily at
the beautiful Fort DeRussy lawn, at the world famous Waikiki Beach in
Honolulu, Hawaii.

Membership is free and open to everyone who wishes to attend any
morning – Monday through Saturday, from 9:00 to 10:30 a.m. for deep
breathing, exercising, meditation, group singing. And on Saturday, after
the class – health lectures on how to live a long, healthy life!

The group averages 75 to 125 per day, according to the seasons. From
December to March it can go up to 200. When away lecturing, their
dedicated leaders carry on until their return. Thousands have visited the
club from around the world and then carry the message of health and fitness
to friends and relatives back home.

Patricia extends an invitation to you and your friends to join the club
for wholesome, healthy fellowship . . . when you visit Honolulu, Hawaii.
Be sure also to visit the outer Hawaiian Islands (Maui, Kauai, Hawaii,
Molakai) for a fulfilling, healthy vacation.

48

HOW TO BEGIN YOUR RUNNING PROGRAM
AND KEEP GOING SUCCESSFULLY

You should get a comfortable pair of shoes with thick rubber soles, particularly under the heel. I often insert foam inner soles, which are carried by most shoe stores. You may feel that the kind of shoes you wear isn't important—but I urge you to take this safeguard of ample padding. Otherwise, the continual jarring of jogging in ill fitting and thin soled shoes could cause eventual discomfort and even total discouragement.

The shoes shouldn't be too loose—or too tight, either. The feet often swell from the added stimulation and circulation during running ... and if the shoes are too tight you'll have established one of the biggest causes of blisters. The same with socks, if you're going to wear them. Make sure they haven't any holes or darns that could cause chafing or blistering ... and make sure they aren't the kind that bunch up inside your shoes. I usually wear two pairs of socks—first a thin pair, then a heavier one, just as many tennis players do.

If you can, *begin your jogging on grass surfaces*. Grass is easier on the legs and feet, especially if you are a big person. The legs are going to do all the harder work and they deserve every consideration you can give them until they are toughened up. Breaking yourself in on grass will give the muscles and joints the chance to loosen up and strengthen themselves.

There will be discomfort—make no mistake about that—particularly if your exercise during the past years has been mostly confined to lifting knife and fork. So, in addition, you need strength of mind to keep at it during the initial periods when progress might be hindered by unexpected and unaccustomed aches, pains and blisters. This soreness is often a healthy sign that changes for the better are underway in your body. Look at it this way, and you'll even take pride in feeling stiff for a few days.

The big rule to follow is TRAIN BUT DON'T STRAIN.

49

ALTERNATE RUNNING AND WALKING

Remember the old Chinese proverb: *"One step is the beginning of a ten thousand mile journey."* Start your new, exciting journey toward Heart Fitness.

One yard is approximately the longest step you can take. Now, step off 25 yards ... or 50 yards ... or 75 or 100. Any one of these distances can be your initial run. If you have not been exercising, make your first run 25 to 50 yards.

Run or jog whatever distance you choose as a starter. After you have made the run, walk three times this distance. Walk briskly, breathing deeply, head up, shoulders back, arms swinging. Deep breathing is important. Remember the reason you are doing this exercise is to give your heart more oxygen.

When you jog every day, the sustained pressure on the circulatory system adds elasticity to the blood vessels, increases their contracted capacity and therefore permits a greater and easier flow of blood. A simple thing ... but a positive step toward ridding yourself of unwanted cholesterol.

One great heart specialist in London told me that any person who will jog 15 to 30 minutes daily for a year could expect to double the capacity of their main arteries. *This is the way to build a powerful heart.*

Activity-breathing (walking, jogging, running, etc.) requires more energy. The body produces this energy by burning foodstuffs, and the burning agent is oxygen. The body can store food at each meal, using what it wants and saving some of the rest for later—but it can't store oxygen.

Most of us produce enough energy to perform ordinary daily activities, but as they become more vigorous, the unfit just can't keep up. This is because, in some bodies, the means for the delivery of oxygen is limited. This is what separates the fit from the unfit.

Jogging and running demands you to breathe more oxygen in and forces your body to process and deliver it. Even if you have been inactive or sick, simple walking and light exercise will soon help you to better circulation and a more vital oxygen intake.

A sound heart, like a sound car, can be driven far and fast without harm . . . but periods of rest and recovery are needed. As we live longer this need generally increases, but not as much as most people imagine. Like that sound car, regular maintenance and sensible use can keep the heart functioning in an "as new" condition even when it's reached vintage age.

I come in the vintage class, as I am more than three score and ten. But I keep running every day and my heart gets stronger and stronger. I start my running program each day by running 100 yards . . . then I walk 100 yards . . . and run 100 yards again. After I get warmed up I run 200 yards . . . then 300 and 400 . . . always walking the same distance I run. This kind of running never puts a strain on my heart.

THE SECRET OF A STRONG HEART
IS GOOD CIRCULATION

When any part of the circulatory system is seriously impaired, the billions of body cells it serves are deprived of their oxygen and nourishment. With their blood supply cut off, these cells will automatically break down. The damage may occur in the heart itself, in the brain, the lungs, kidneys, skin or other parts of the body.

Just remember . . . if you do not use the body you lose it!

5 EXERCISES FOR SPEEDING UP CIRCULATION

Exercise No. 1—The Windmill Exercise

(A) Stand erect with heels and toes together, chest up, abdomen drawn in, shoulders back, head high, chin in, hands hanging loosely at sides. Now start a circular motion foward, the hands and arms making a complete circle forward along the sides of the body. Increase the speed until you are making circles as fast as possible. Start doing 10 circles forward and increase by several a day until you can bring it up to 50 circles at one time.

(B) Same position as Exercise No. 1 (A), only instead of making circles with the hands forward, make circles backward —in the opposite direction.

Exercise No. 2—Circulation-Builder

(This exercise is the same as is used by people in cold climates who want to bring circulation to their arms, hands and upper body.)

Same position as Exercise No. 1. Arms and hands outstretched horizontally at shoulder height. Each hand forms a half circle as the exercise is done. The right hand strikes the left shoulder and the left hand strikes the right shoulder at the same time, and then alternately. The arms are crisscrossed alternately ... right over left, left over right ... (repeating), and slap the shoulders vigorously. I repeat, make it vigorous so that each time the arms are flung open back to starting-position the chest is pushed forward. Start this exercise by doing it 10 times and work up until you can do it 50 times.

Exercise No. 3—The Leg and Foot Vibrating-Exercise

Stand erect, feet about 8 to 10 inches apart, arms at sides. Now put all your weight on the left foot and raise your right foot off the ground about 6 or 8 inches. Make short kicks (4 to 5 inches) in a forward direction, as hard as possible. The leg should be vibrated from the hips to the toes. Now alternate, standing on right foot, kicking the left foot. Start with 10 kicks on each foot and increase the amount every day until you can kick about 50 times or more, each foot. Make this a vigorous action as it will promote great circulation to the hip, thigh, calf and foot.

Exercise No. 4—Promoting Circulation in Hands and Fingers

Stand erect as in Position No. 1. Bring the hands about 10 inches in front of the body, chest height, and from the wrists violently shake the relaxed hands. I repeat, be sure that the hand is relaxed and shake it violently from the wrist. Do 15 hard shakes with both hands at the same time and then grip the hands hard 15 times ... grip each hand individually into a tight fist, then relax it, extending the fingers out as far as possible.

52

Exercise No. 5—Exercise for Blood Circulation in Head

Stand erect with feet about 12 inches apart. Lean forward from the waist, with arms hanging loosely and relaxed in front as near to the floor as possible. In this position violently shake the head from side to side and forward to back. Do this exercise only a few times in the beginning, until your head becomes accustomed to the stimulated circulation.

NO HEART STRAIN FROM EXERCISE

These exercises are ideal for speeding up circulation and opening up blocked arteries and other blood vessels. When the circulation is increased through exercise, the blood is purified in the lungs and oxygen is carried to all parts of the body.

A normal, healthy heart cannot be injured by these exercises, regardless of how long or how strenuously you do them. Weak persons should start slowly, and work up to a vigorous performance. These circulatory exercises are beneficial not only to a normal but to an injured heart as well, just as to any other muscle. They condition your heart just as they do your visible muscles.

Refuse to listen to people who try to frighten you away from exercise! *The heart is a muscle and must be exercised,* if it is to remain strong. By exercising you are building a vigorous, strong heart and body!

Every one of these exercises should be done daily. This will require about 15 to 20 minutes—little enough time to invest in a healthy heart and a healthful life! If you have a sedentary position ... if you spend a lot of time sitting or standing ... you should do these exercises 2 or 3 times every day. When you are on a long automobile drive, stop and take these circulatory exercises every hour. The more you do these exercises, the better circulation you will have ... and better circulation means a stronger heart!

When at home, follow this exercise period with the Special Bath, as described in the following instructions.

Difficulties strengthen the mind as labor does the body.

SPECIAL BATHING INSTRUCTIONS
FOR BETTER CIRCULATION

This is a progressive method for improving the circulation over the entire body. Your equipment includes a large back brush or Swedish bath friction mitt, a cake of good, imported castile soap, and a large, coarse Turkish towel.

Get into the shower bath and turn on the hot water. Make it as hot as you can comfortably take it. Now with soap and brush or mitt, scrub your body thoroughly. At first your coddled body will not be able to take much pressure from the brush or mitt . . . so go lightly! As you condition your skin to vigorous workouts, however, it will be able to take an enormous amount of scrubbing.

After you have washed your body thoroughly in hot water, start cooling the water down . . . cooler and cooler to the coolest temperature you can possibly stand without feeling a shock or too great a reaction.

For wonderful relaxation of tired muscles and refreshing stimulation, alternate the hot and cold water several times, letting the shower spray beat heavily on back and shoulders. I advise business people on days when they come home tense and tired to take this relaxing shower before dinner. They find it makes them refreshed and relaxed.

TRAINING THE BODY—NOT STRAINING

Remember this is a progressive method, to be accomplished slowly over a period of time . . . each time making the water a little hotter and a little colder . . . but never beyond your body's tolerance. *I do not believe in straining the body, but in conditioning and training it.* This hot-and-cold shower is a marvelous heart-and-circulation conditioner, because you push your heart and circulatory system to the limit by forcing yourself to take water as hot as you can stand and as cold as you can stand. The hotter and the colder you can take it, the more fit your heart will become and the better will be your circulation.

After you have soaped and showered with hot water and turned on the cold water, rinse all the soap from the brush or mitt and start rubbing your body all over as the cold water hits it. Each day increase the vigor with which you rub your body.

As you feel the tingle of exhilarated circulation, step out of the shower, get a large, coarse Turkish towel that is new (when they get too soft pass them on to the delicate members of the family). Now take this large, coarse Turkish towel and for 10 minutes rub and towel every inch of your body from head to toe.

When you have gone through this Special Bath every day for one year, you will be ready to graduate to the Polar Bear Club. The members of the Polar Bear Club do not use towels on the wet body—only on the dry body. After the hot-and-cold shower with its vigorous brushing, dry your body with vigorous hand rubbing. Only after you have dried yourself with your hands do you take the towel. Now rub yourself with your extra-heavy coarse towel for an additional 10 minutes. The circulation will go whirling through your body!

EXERCISE TO IMPROVE THE KIDNEYS

The kidneys of the body are the great filters. They are the hardest working organs in the body. Exercises that bend and twist the body at its middle help to stimulate the kidneys and they function more efficiently.

There is no better exercise for stimulating the kidneys than this one:

Stand up straight with hands over head. Now bend forward from the waist and try to touch the toes without bending the knees. Return hands over head, then bend backwards as far as possible.

Another good exercise to strengthen the kidneys is to clasp the hands over the head, then bend first to the left side and then to the right side as far as possible.

Since most of the body's waste products are eliminated through the kidneys, you should do these kidney stimulating exercises daily . . . starting with 10 times and working up to 50 times for each exercise.

He who cannot find time for exercise, will have to find time for illness.
—Lord Derby

THE DANGERS OF SITTING TOO LONG

Although most waste products are eliminated through the kidneys, carbon dioxide is expelled from the body through the lungs. There the blood takes on a fresh supply of oxygen and again turns a bright red. It then flows back into the heart, to be pumped out through the arteries to the rest of the body. This powerful cycle is repeated thousands of time a day.

That is the reason you must never sit too long at one time. *Sitting slows down the circulation and stagnates the blood.* Long periods of sitting or inactivity could of course, damage the heart. Man was never made to be a sedentary creature.

People who sit too long may develop a thrombosis (blood clot) in the deep veins of the calf. If your work in an office requires a lot of sitting, *get up and move around every hour.* When you take a long automobile trip, make it a point to stop the car every hour on the hour and get out and take a good, brisk walk or do the circulatory exercises as noted earlier. Remember when you exercise you are flushing poisons out of the cells of the body and renewing the vital circulation of blood through the hundreds of miles of "pipes" that supply these cells with food and oxygen.

HOW TO SIT

If you have to sit—sit correctly! The most disastrous and *injurious habit is crossing the legs.* Don't sit with your legs crossed! Crossing the legs can compress the popliteal artery (in back of the knees) and may also be a cause of stagnation in the veins.

When you sit in a chair sit well back. Do not let the edge of the chair cut off the circulation in back of the knees. Keep your feet on the floor. Dangling your legs puts too much pressure on the veins. When my children were small, I cut down a table by sawing off the legs, so that when the children sat at it their feet would touch the floor. Adults who are short in stature should use a footstool.

A rocker is the best type of chair to sit in. You can get your rest by sitting . . . and some exercise by rocking!

56

SWEAT FOR HEALTH

The skin, with its millions of pores and sweat glands, is the largest eliminating organ of the body. Sweat has a dual purpose ... it helps rid the body of impurities ... and it serves as a temperature regulator. When our body is exposed to heat or is "warmed up" by exercise, the sweat glands are stimulated into action. Evaporation of the sweat cools the blood when it reaches the skin and thus helps to prevent the body from becoming overheated, and at the same time impurities near the surface are eliminated.

It is these impurities, or the mixture with dirt on the skin, which gives sweat an unpleasant odor. If you are clean inside and out, there is only the good smell of "honest sweat." And regardless of what deodorant advertisers say, *it is healthy to sweat.*

Dancing, walking, bicycling, vigorous housework . . . any kind of activity that will make you sweat improves your heart action and your general health. Hard work never hurt anyone!

INDULGE IN HOBBIES THAT ARE ACTIVE

If I were the President of the United States I would advocate laws that would require all people who sit down and play cards to spend an equal amount of time in keeping physically fit by brisk walking. The same for the "idiot box" (television) addict. For every hour he sits before this contraption he would have to spend an hour in brisk walking.

I would start a crusade against inactivity, long sitting and sedentary activities. Sitting slows down the circulation, and when the circulation is slowed down many changes take place in the artery walls. You must keep active. When you relax, relax actively. Cultivate hobbies that give you needed exercise ... exercise that you enjoy, such as hiking, swimming, tennis, golf. You cannot build a strong heart unless you walk briskly, bend, twist and vibrate your body so that your blood is moving swiftly through it.

Our days are identical suitcases—all the same size, but some people can pack more into them than others.

57

DO NOT WEAR CONSTRICTING GARMENTS

Anything that impedes the circulation of the blood damages the heart. Therefore, there should be no constricting garments on our body. This includes tight garters, foundation garments that constrict rather than support, tight belts, tight collars and ties . . . and above all, tight shoes.

NO BINDING SHOES

Tight shoes can do more to disturb the circulation than any other article of clothing, because the feet must always be well supplied with blood. There are 26 bones in each foot—more than in any other part of the body. When the blood does not reach the feet in the required quantities, poisons are retained in the cell structures of the feet. That is why many feet have an unpleasant odor.

Many conditions of stiffness and deformities are brought on by ill-fitting shoes which cause poor circulation and incorrect posture in walking and standing. Shoes must be worn that do not bind or inhibit the free circulation of the blood to the feet.

Walking barefoot is the ideal way to walk. Every opportunity we have to take off our shoes and walk barefoot means that we are improving our circulation and working toward the fitness of our heart. Walking on the grass, walking on the earth, or simply walking barefoot around the house improves the circulation and helps strengthen the heart.

HOW TO BUILD BETTER CIRCULATION
IN THE EXTREMETIES OF YOUR BODY

The heart must pump blood to the legs and feet, as well as to the hands. Most persons do not have sufficient rhythmic circulation to these extremities, and that is why so many people complain of cold feet, numb feet, legs that "go to sleep" easily, arms and hands that become numb.

There is a hydrotherapeutic method to alleviate these conditions by stimulating the circulation. It is known as the *Cold and Hot Method.*

58

Get two small foot tubs or wash tubs. Fill one with hot water about 104° or as hot as you can stand. Fill the other with cold water, preferably with ice cubes added.

Now stand for 2 minutes with your feet in the hot water and your hands and arms (up to the elbows) submerged in the cold water. After 2 minutes, reverse the procedure—put the feet in the cold water and the arms and hands in the hot water for 2 minutes. Repeat this five times, then take a coarse towel and rub feet, arms and hands vigorously until they have a pinkish glow.

A SOUND MIND IN A SOUND BODY

It was Shakespeare who anticipated by many years the dominant psychology of our time when he said, "It is the mind that makes a body rich."

True it is that mind helps body . . . likewise, body helps mind.

We have a twofold relationship with the Universe—and this we must never forget except to our loss. We are related to the Infinite Spirit of Life . . . the life and the power in the Universe . . . in that it is the life within us—our very own life. In order to experience life in its fullness, we must live continually in this realization. This is the mental, the spiritual, the soul life.

We also have the life of the body which relates us to this particular portion of the Universe on which we live . . . the Earth, we call it. We are related to Mother Earth through the food we eat, the water we drink, the air we breathe, the sun with its all-pervading power. All these are essential not only to a healthy body, but to the very continuance of our life and body here. These we must get in the purity as Nature provides them, without depleting them—or de-naturing them, as we say.

Take the food we eat, for example, which is intimately related to health or its opposite. It is the bloodstream with its marvelous distribution system which carries the essentials that provide the energy and vitality for the functioning of

59

every part of the body. And what we eat at this hour today will be in our bloodstream within 24 hours.

If we eat the food as Nature herself prepared it with her own unmatched chemistry ... without its being de-natured of essential elements ... then it will meet every requirement for healthy growth and chemical balance of the body. It will build you a powerful and long lasting heart. It will give you an alert and active mind. It will add life to your years—and years to your life!

YOU ARE WHAT YOU EAT

A couple of generations ago the main elements of food were known only as *proteins, fats and carbohydrates*—the primary building and fuel supplies of the body. Since then, however, Nutritional Science has discovered that Nature also provides various regulating agents—*minerals, vitamins and chemicals* —which are equally essential for the healthy and harmonious functioning of the body.

No one can be healthy if this balance is disturbed. Yet it is constantly being tampered with. To give foods a longer "shelf life" in the markets, certain elements are depleted and/or certain preservatives added—thus changing the natural content of the food. These de-natured foods—and natural foods as well—are further devitalized by improper methods of preparing and cooking.

It has truly been said that *"Americans are the most overfed and undernourished people in the world."* And this is the main reason why the No. 1 Killer—Heart Attack—is having a field day in the United States!

ARE YOU POISONING YOUR BODY?

If you are eating the kind of food that most Americans and people of other affluent, industralized countries are eating, you are slowly but surely poisoning yourself. You are filling yourself with foodless foods ... and depriving your body of the natural foods that it needs. And you may also be among the many who are hastening this suicidal process by adding such toxic poisons as tobacco, alcohol, coffee, tea and cola drinks.

60

There is a great deal of discussion today about polluted air and polluted water. But what about a polluted bloodstream? Here is something which you, as an individual, can do something about. You can start today to detoxicate your body!

Eliminate the following materials from your diet—and you will eliminate the No. 1 Killer, Heart Attack. Heart Attack cannot deliver the fatal blow unless your body is already weakened by this gang of poisoners. Post this in your kitchen —and keep them out of your bloodstream!

WANTED
FOR MURDER

KILLER Saturated Fat
CHOKER Hydrogenated Fat
CLOGGER Salt
DEADEYED Devitalized Foods
DOPEY Caffeine
HARD Water
PLUGGER Frying Pan
CRAZY Alcohol
SMOKEY Tobacco
JERKEY Turbulent Emotions
LOAFER Laziness
GREASY Overweight
HOGGY Over-Eating

DON'T CLOSE THE ARTERIES WITH THE RESIDUE OF TOBACCO, ALCOHOL, COFFEE, TEA, COLA DRINKS, SALT AND SATURATED FATS!

It is impossible to have smooth, flexible arteries through which the oxygen-enriched blood can flow freely—when you allow these poisons to enter your body. The tars and chemicals from tobacco leave a poisonous residue on the walls of the arteries . . . and the same thing may be said against tea, coffee, cola drinks and saturated fats.

Not only do these poisons clog your arteries. Tobacco, coffee, tea, alcohol and cola drinks are also powerful stimulants to the heart. The heart has a normal rhythm which it can maintain indefinitely under healthful conditions. But when you use these harsh stimulants, you actually whip and beat your heart into unnatural activity that causes it to be overworked.

TOBACCO IN ANY FORM IS AN ENEMY OF THE HEART

Whether in cigarets, cigars or pipes, tobacco is one of the heart's greatest enemies. Here is what *Dr. Lester M. Morrison,* noted Los Angeles heart specialist and pioneer in the low-cholesterol diet for the treatment and prevention of heart disease, has to say about tobacco:

"Tobacco is a poison ... Nicotine, one of the main ingredients of tobacco, is a poison affecting the brain, the heart and other vital organs. The tobacco plant is directly related to the deadly nightshade family of plants ... Aside from the *chief poison, nicotine,* there are other wellknown poisons present in tobacco: *carbon monoxide* (when tobacco is burned), *arsenic* and *coal tar* substances are some." Dr. Morrison also notes, *"Nicotine is the most noxious substance than can affect the blood vessels in man."*

Nicotine is a powerful drug that constricts the arteries, narrowing still more these vital passageways of the blood, which have been clogged by other toxic residue. The tobacco smoker does double damage to his heart—first, by filling the bloodstream with the harsh poisons of tobacco, and second, by narrowing the arteries and other blood vessels, thus preventing a free flow of life giving blood.

The body has no defense against the carbon monoxide produced by smoking. You have read about people committing suicide or being killed by carbon monoxide fumes. Why deliberately breathe them into your lungs?

The coal tars in tobacco are the poisons which have been found to be chiefly responsible for cancer of the lungs, mouth and related areas of the body.

It frightens me to think of what is going to happen in another 25 years of the excessive use of tobacco. I am convinced that every smoker will develop *lung cancer*—unless *heart disease* or some other fatal illness claims him earlier!

SMOKING AND EMPHYSEMA GO HAND IN HAND

Another killer disease that comes from smoking is emphysema, which is greatly on the increase today. In fact, a recent report from medical authorities in Washington shows that as many as half of all adult American men are suffering to some degree from emphysema.

In this disease the tars, nicotine and other destructive poisons of tobacco lodge in the small air sacs of the lungs, causing the sac walls to become very thin or to break down entirely, so that the blood is no longer able to exchange poisonous carbon dioxide for life-giving oxygen. The victim dies of oxygen starvation . . . he is slowly smothered to death from within.

Emphysema is not a quick killer. It creeps up on a smoker. At first there is a slight cough especially on arising . . . then it becomes a cough that plagues the smoker day and night. Slowly but surely the air sacs of the lungs are almost completely destroyed. The victim does not die suddenly, but lingers on in a steadily deteriorating condition. He is forced to be near an oxygen tank because the disease is shutting off his supply of life-giving oxygen. Finally, when the lungs cannot operate any longer even to take in pure oxygen, the victim dies.

Our breath is our life. We can live days without water and weeks without food . . . but we can live only minutes without air. Air is the very first essential in our existence. And it is the oxygen in the air we breathe that is the greatest purifying force in Nature . . . to get this oxygen into the lungs and the bloodstream, we must breathe it in.

Smoking tobacco is against every Natural Law . . . and when you attempt to break a Law of Nature, the Law will break YOU. *The heart needs a large amount of oxygen to function.* Any disease that diminishes the supply of oxygen is going to destroy the health of your heart, lungs and entire body.

Open thou mine eyes, that I may behold wondrous things out of thy law. —Psalm 119:18

SMOKING ROBS YOUR BODY OF VITAMIN C

Vitamin C is one of Nature's essential elements for good health. In addition to its other important functions—such as the prevention of scurvy—*Vitamin C is also active in preventing hemorrhaging of the capillaries,* those tiny blood vessels that directly feed the cells of the body.

When the capillaries in the artery walls hemorrhage, it causes additional blockage to the flow of the mainstream of the blood. When this occurs in the heart or the brain, a serious clot may form. In the hands and feet serious breakdown of the capillaries may occur, sometimes causing gangrene that may result in an amputation. *

So you can see how essential Vitamin C is to the healthy functioning of your heart and bloodstream and your entire body.

Tobacco neutralizes Vitamin C in your body—robbing you of this vital protection. *Dr. W. J. McCormick,* Vitamin C specialist of Canada, found in laboratory and clinical tests that *the smoking of a single cigaret robs the body of the amount of Vitamin C* contained in one medium sized orange. A "pack a day" smoker would have to consume 20 oranges in order to maintain a normal balance of essential Vitamin C in his body!

Tobacco is not the only robber of Vitamin C. The *polluted air* of our cities and the foods which contain *chemical preservatives also exhaust this essential vitamin.*

STOP SMOKING TODAY!

Many smokers are so addicted to this unhealthy and filthy habit that they are cry babies and say, "It's impossible for me to break the habit of smoking."

All I say is, "Rubbish! *Who controls your body—the tobacco or you?*" Flesh is dumb. It has no intelligence. You must control the body with the mind. The mind should always force the body to obey its orders.

---

* *Cigerette smokers have 50% higher atherosclerosis and hypertension deaths!*

In my lecture work all over the world I have had health *students in my classes who have smoked for as many as 50 years—and they stopped without tapering off.* They made up their minds to stop smoking at once—and they did.

Of course, they suffered for a few days. Of course their nerves cried out for the nicotine "dope" of the tobacco. But they had the intenstinal fortitude to take the punishment of the withdrawal discomforts. They were fighting a vicious monster that had controlled them. They won their battle.

THE POWER OF DEEP DESIRE

To be effective in *changing a bad habit into a good one, rational thought must be accompanied by deep feeling and desire. If you desire a Healthy Heart strongly enough, you can conquer the tobacco habit.*

Picture yourself as you would like to be, and assume for the moment that such a thing might be possible. In forming good habits and breaking bad ones, we have to deal with *thought habits.* "As a man thinketh in his heart, so is he." Think, "NO SMOKING!" Tell yourself over and over that smoking is slowly killing you, and it is your bitter enemy. Say to yourself over and over again, "Tobacco in any form is a killer —and I am through with the vicious poison forever."

Repeat, "I will not smoke! I will not smoke! I will not smoke!" You will become a master over your body instead of a slave to tobacco.

You must not be a slave to any bad habit that is damaging your heart and body, and that might bring on a heart attack. That goes not only for tobacco—but for coffee, tea, alcohol, salt and saturated fats.

Free yourself from the bondage of these killing habits. Look upon all these poisons as your enemies. To have a strong, healthy heart you must systematically practice "Health Mindedness." In your mind's eye see yourself as you wish to be— strong and healthy and youthful . . . a person who is complete master of his body . . . not a grovelling slave to any life destroying habit.

Habits that destroy the health and the body must be broken with a willpower that is stronger than the bad habit.

SAY TO YOURSELF:

- "I will not use tobacco."
- "I will not drink coffee."
- "I will not drink tea."
- "I will not use salt."
- "I will not over-eat."
- "I will not drink colas."
- "I will not drink alcoholic drinks."
- "I will not overburden my body with saturated fats."

Say to yourself over and over—and believe it! that your intelligent mind will control your body.

Let no one or no circumstance break your iron willpower. Let no one brainwash you. You do your own thinking. You control your own mind and body. This is how you break bad habits of any kind.

COFFEE AND TEA ARE DRUGS *

Coffee is a powerful, harmful stimulant to the heart. It contains the drug caffeine which makes the heart beat faster and puts an undue strain upon it. Coffee also contains tars and acids which are injurious to the heart and blood vessels and other tissues, and these are also present in de-caffeinated coffee. Keep all kinds of coffee away from the table! It has no nutrients, no vitamins and minerals. It is worthless as a food —and harmful to your health.

The same goes for tea. It contains tannic acid and other toxic substances. Don't contaminate your bloodstream.

COLA DRINKS ARE TOXIC

What do cola drinks consist of? Three toxic stimulants and carbonated water! Colas contain caffeine, phosphoric acid and refined white sugar ... nothing but "empty calories" without any nutrient value ... plus the irritating effects of the carbonated water on the kidneys and liver ... plus the poisons in the drugs. Don't drink colas—and don't let your children ruin their health with these drinks!

---

* *Coffee increases free fatty acid levels in the blood and causes degenerative diseases! ''There is a strong likelihood that caffeine may prove to be one of the most dangerous mutagens in man,''*   Cancer Research Nov. 1968

Dangerous Habit: How much coffee do you drink? A recent survey found that 17% of American's have one cup a day, 15% two cups, 10% three cups, 7% four cups, 12% five or more cups, and 38% none at all. Coffee ia a "no-no" for health!

ALCOHOL IS A DEPRESSANT

Although it is generally considered a stimulant, alcohol is actually a depressant. It dilates the blood vessels, especially the capillaries in the skin, and thus gives a sensation of warmth that is mistaken for being stimulated or "pepped up." As a matter of fact, the opposite is taking place. Alcohol is a relaxant—and it can be so relaxing that one loses all control of one's actions. Who hasn't seen a drunk so "relaxed" that he topples into the gutter? *Drinking alcohol is a dangerous way to relax!*

The chief *toxic effect* of alcohol is on *the brain and nervous system.* Alcohol "burns up" or *depletes the body of both Vitamin C and Vitamin B,* the essential "nerve vitamin." Hemorrhages that occur in the brain often result in paralysis. In fact, medical research has shown that the boisterous actions —the loud speech, the "hail-fellow-well-met" joviality—of the alcoholic, his bravado and devil-may-care attitude, are actually *the results of a beginning paralysis of certain parts of the brain.*

Stay away from alcohol! It has nothing but *"empty calories"* that will burden your body with unhealthy, flabby fat . . . plus its other poisonous and injurious effects.

Of *special danger to anyone with a heart condition* is the numbing effect of alcohol on the pain centers of the brain and nervous system. Without Nature's warning signal—pain—a heart attack which might have been averted may prove fatal.

"KILLER" FOODS

If drink can kill—so can food. Don't dig your grave with your teeth!

To have a heart that is fit, your blood chemistry must be balanced. The 8 quarts of blood in your body must have all of the *60 nutrients that build a powerful, fit heart.*

Once there was a time when man did not need to know what to leave out of his diet. That was because the only foods that he had to eat were those that Nature produced. They were not robbed of their natural elements as they are today.

AVOID THESE PROCESSED, REFINED, HARMFUL FOODS

Once you realize the irreparable harm caused to your body by refined, chemicalized, deficient foods, it is not difficult to eat correctly. Simply eliminate these "killer" foods from your diet...and follow an eating plan which provides the basic, essential nourishment your body needs.

- Refined sugar or refined sugar products such as jams, jellies, preserves, marmalades, yogurts, ice cream, sherberts, Jello, cake, candy, cookies, chewing gum, soft drinks, pies, pastries, tapioca puddings, sugared fruit juices & fruits canned in sugar syrup.

- Salted foods, such as corn chips, salted crackers, salted nuts

- Catsup & mustard w/salt-sugar, Worchestershire sauce, pickles, olives

- White rice & pearled barley   • Fried & greasy foods

- Commercial, highly processed dry cereals such as corn flakes, etc.

- Saturated fats & hydrogenated oils...(heart enemies that clog bloodstream)

- Food which contains palm & cottonseed oil. Products labeled vegetable oil...find out what kind, before you use it.

- Oleo & margarines...(saturated fats & hydrogenated oils)

- Peanut butter that contains hydrogenated, hardened oils

- Coffee, decaffeinated coffee, China black tea & all alcoholic beverages

- Fresh pork & pork products   • Fried, fatty & greasy meats

- Smoked meats, such as ham, bacon & sausage, smoked fish

- Luncheon meats, such as hot dogs, salami, bologna, corned beef, pastrami & any packaged meats containing dangerous sodium nitrate or nitrite

- Dried fruits containing sulphur dioxide - a preservative

- Do not eat chickens that have been injected with stilbestrol, or fed with chicken feed that contains any drug

- Canned soups - read labels for sugar, starch, white, wheat flour & preservatives

- Food that contains benzoate of soda, salt, sugar, cream of tartar...& any additives, drugs or preservatives

- White flour products such as white bread, wheat-white bread, enriched flours, rye bread that has wheat-white flour in it, dumplings, biscuits, buns, gravy, noodles, pancakes, waffles, soda crackers, macaroni, spaghetti, pizza, ravioli, pies, pastries, cakes, cookies , prepared and commercial puddings, and ready-mix bakery products. (Health Stores have a huge variety of 100% whole grain products.)

- Day-old, cooked vegetables & potatoes, & pre-mixed old salads

FOOD AND PRODUCT SUMMARY

Today many of our foods are highly processed or refined, thus robbing them of essential nutrients, vitamins, minerals, and enzymes; many contain harmful and dangerous chemicals.

The research, findings, and experience of top nutritionists, physicians and dentists have led them to discover that devitalized foods are a major cause of poor health, illness, cancer and premature death. The enormous increase in the last seventy years in degenerative diseases such as heart disease, arthritis, and dental decay, would seem to substantiate this belief. Scientific research has shown most of these afflictions may be prevented; and others, when once established, may be arrested or in some cases even reversed through nutritional methods.

THESE STEPS ARE FOR SUPER HEALTH THROUGH HEALTHY, WHOLESOME, NATURAL FOOD

1. Serve foods in raw, original state, organically grown when possible – fresh fruits, vegetables, wholegrains, brown rice, beans, raw nuts & seeds.

2. PROTEIN

   a. Animal meat, including the variety meats — liver, kidney, brain, heart — poultry and sea food, suggest using sparingly. Cook meat as little as possible (bake, roast, wok, or broil) because protein is injured by prolonged high heat. (My Dad and I prefer a vegetarian diet.)

   b. Dairy products, eggs (fertile), unprocessed hard cheese, and certified raw milk. (Personally we do not use milk and only occasionally low-fat dairy by-products).

   c. The legumes, soy and all other beans . . . these are our favorites.

   d. Nuts and seeds, raw and unsalted.

3. Use FRUITS and VEGETABLES (organically grown without the use of poisonous chemical sprays and fertilizers, when possible). Ask your market to stock organic produce. Steam, bake, saute or wok vegetables with a minimum of distilled water, at low heat, for as short a time as possible. Use the vegetable liquid.

4. Use 100% WHOLEGRAIN CEREALS, BREADS, & FLOURS, they contain important B complex vitamins, vitamin E, minerals, & the important unsaturated fatty acids.

5. Use COLD-PROCESSED VEGETABLE OILS, OLIVE OIL, CANOLA and SESAME OIL, etc.... These are an excellent source of the healthy essential unsaturated fatty acids, but still use sparingly.

4 BRAGG BOOKS FOR PLANNING HEALTHY MEALS

These Books are a must reading for planning your Bragg Health Building Program. They are: • *Healthful Eating Without Confusion* • *Bragg's Health Gourmet Recipes For Vital Healthy Living* (448 pages) • *Bragg Vegetarian Health Gourmet Recipes* (sugar free, salt free, low fat) and the • *Bragg Health Sauerkraut (raw, salt free) Recipe Book* ... Learn why and how to make your own delicious sauerkraut – it's so healthy for you. See back pages for ordering.

NO SELF-DRUGGING!

You are not qualified to prescribe drugs for yourself. The results could be serious. So ... no straight Aspirin or products containing Aspirin ... no Anti-histamines ... no Milk of Magnesia ... no sleeping pills, tranquilizers or pain killers ... no strong cathartics or fizzing bromides. Take none of these unless prescribed by your physician, and then follow his directions exactly.

GET IN THE HABIT OF EATING FOR HEALTH

You need to learn not only what to leave out of your diet ... but just as important, *what to put into your diet.* Once you understand the *basic principles of proper nourishment,* the elements your body must have to build, develop and live as it was meant to do naturally ... you will find that you can nourish your body without sacrificing meal-time enjoyment. Combinations of *healthful foods* packed with vital nutrients are almost limitless.

The first step, of course, is to *get into the habit of eating for health.* Such a habit is not difficult to form. Although the instinctive sense of food selection has been submerged because of the artificial character of most foods in popular use today, *this natural sense can be restored* to a great degree by proper eating. Like any other ability or skill, it must be kept constantly in practice or its powers will deteriorate. Only by exercising these powers can we revive and strengthen them.

Degenerative diseases stem from breakdowns from within, not from attacks from without ... although the latter may occur secondarily as a result of weakened defenses.

Since degenerative diseases arise within our bodies because of some lack of vital substance or substances, our safest course is to reinforce our defenses with those elements which will give them the power to resist. *One's body is like a fortress.* Many persons appear alike on the *out*side—but *inside* there may be conditions which make one person strong and another weak. Well-marshaled forces within a fortress can repel the enemy ... poorly organized forces succumb. Let

70

us build our inner strength so that we will be impervious to all deadly enemies of the body.

Let me quote again from the eminent heart specialist, *Dr. Lester Morrison*, who states: "*In the degenerative diseases of the heart and blood vessels, diet is the key; it is the difference between active good health and dangerous illness.*"

KEEP CLEAN INSIDE

To have a clean, healthy bloodstream and arteries free from encrustation and corrosion, we must not only eat correctly but also drink correctly. *The liquids which go into our bodies must be pure and nourishing.*

To begin with, I believe that every person should have the equivalent of *6 to 8 glasses of rain water or distilled water every day.* Rain water is man's ideal drink. It is pure, distilled water coming directly from the heavens above us, through the clear, uncontaminated air thousands of feet above the earth. If we cannot get rain water, we should buy distilled water. It can be obtained in most markets and grocery stores, drug stores or chemist shops. If you cannot find it readily, look under "WATER" or "DISTILLED" in the yellow classified pages of your telephone directory.

Rain water and distilled water have no inorganic minerals to deposit themselves on the walls of the arteries and other "pipes" of the body.

In contrast, *well water, spring water and river water all contain inorganic minerals which cannot under any circumstances be utilized in the body chemistry.* They corrode the human "pipes" just as they do the iron pipes which bring this water into your home.

HARD WATER MAY CAUSE HARDENING OF THE ARTERIES

The human body has a vast pipe system. A healthy heart must have clear coronary arteries. The blood must be able to flow through them smoothly to nourish the heart and keep it pumping steadily and efficiently.

But suppose a person drinks only hard water (as most people do) and the pipelines become clogged and blocked with inorganic minerals which cannot be absorbed into the body? Blockage in the coronary arteries that feed the heart means that the amount of blood reaching the heart muscles is reduced. When the blood supply is reduced below a certain point, the affected parts of the heart muscles can no longer function. *When a section of heart muscle stops functioning a heart attack and even death may result.*

This blockage occurs not only in the arteries of the heart itself, but it can happen throughout the arterial pipelines. If it occurs in the arteries going into the brain, serious damage can be done and paralysis may be the result.

Arteriosclerosis or hardening of the arteries means that the arteries have become brittle and lost their elasticity, due to injurious deposits in the artery walls. The entire pipe system may become so blocked that the blood, carrying oxygen and nourishment to the cells of the body and its vital organs, cannot get through . . . or that the flow which does get through is insufficient.

Most people want to blame hardening of the arteries on their calendar years. But calendar years do not put inorganic minerals into the arteries. *Time is not toxic* . . . time is not a force that damages the body. Time is a measure and nothing else. *Don't blame your years for your physical troubles!* You can only blame yourself for not taking care of this wonderful body with which Nature equipped you.

THE DIFFERENCE BETWEEN ORGANIC AND INORGANIC MINERALS

Inorganic minerals are inert . . . which means that they *cannot be absorbed into the body.*

Organic minerals are those which come from that which is *living* or has lived . . . and *16 of these organic minerals are essential elements of the human body.* When we eat an apple or any other fruit or vegetable, that substance is living, for it has a certain length of life after it has been picked. The same is true for animals foods, fish, milk, cheese and eggs. Animals obtain their organic minerals from plants. We humans obtain our organic minerals from both plants and animals.

Only the living plant has the power to.extract inorganic minerals from the earth and change them into organic minerals. No animal or human can do this. If you were cast away on an uninhabited island where nothing was growing you would starve to death. Although the soil beneath your feet would contain 16 inorganic minerals, your body could not absorb them.

Organic minerals are vital in keeping us alive and healthy . . . but inorganic minerals can kill us.

Many years ago I was on an expedition in China, when one part of the country was suffering from drought and famine. I saw with my own eyes . . . poor, starving people heating dirt and eating it, for want of food. They died horrible deaths, because they could not get one bit of nourishment from the inorganic minerals of the earth.

INORGANIC MINERALS IN WATER
ARE HARMFUL TO HEALTH

For years I have heard people say that certain waters were rich in all the minerals. What minerals are they talking about? Inorganic or organic? They are simply burdening their bodies with these inert minerals, which may cause the development of stones in the kidneys and gall bladder and acid crystals in the arteries, veins, joints, and other parts of the body.

I was reared in a part of Virginia where the drinking water is called "hard water." It is heavily saturated with inorganic minerals, especially sodium, iron and calcium. I saw many of my adult relations and friends die of kidney troubles. Nearly all of the people were prematurely old, because the inorganic minerals would collect on the inner walls of the arteries and veins, causing them to die with hardening of the arteries. One of my uncles died at the great Johns Hopkins Hospital in Baltimore, Maryland, when he was only 48 years of age. The doctors who performed the autopsy after death stated that his arteries were as hard as clay pipes, because they were so corroded with inorganic minerals.

Little things are like weeds—-the longer we neglect them, the larger they grow.

RAIN AND FRUIT JUICES ARE
NATURE'S DISTILLED WATER

No new water has been put on the face of the earth since it was originally formed. Just as the same energy is formed and re-formed, so the same water is usable over and over again by the miracle of Nature. Waters of the earth are *purified by distillation.* The sun evaporates the water ... it is collected into clouds and the clouds become full and then we have rain and dew ... pure, perfectly clean water ... *absolutely free of all harmful inorganic substances.*

Years ago, when the late Douglas Fairbanks, Senior, and I were close friends, we roamed the South Sea Islands for several months. During that trip we came upon an island inhabited by *beautiful, healthy Polynesians* who never drank any water but distilled water, because the island was surrounded by the Pacific Ocean. This sea water was undrinkable because of the high salt content. Their island was based on porous coral which could not hold water ... so they would *only drink rain water,* or the fresh, clear, clean water of the green coconut. I have never seen any finer specimens of men or women than these native South Sea Islanders. There were several doctors on the yacht who thoroughly examined the oldest people on these islands, and one heart doctor stated that he had never examined such well-preserved people in his life.

You noted that I said only the most mature people were examined by our doctors ... *they were completely unaware of age* because no such word existed in their language. They never celebrated birthdays, so they were gloriously ageless ... not only in years but in body. These older men performed as well in the vigorous native dances as the younger men. They were beautiful specimens of manhood and womanhood, and they had lived their lengthy lives drinking only Nature's distilled water.

If you drink rain water or snow water, or the fresh juices of fruits and vegetables, remember that all of this liquid has been *distilled by Nature.*

Rain water and snow water are 100% mineral-free.

Fresh fruit and vegetable juices contain Nature's pure *distilled water*, plus certain nutrients such as *natural sugar, organic minerals* and *vitamins*.

WHY I DRINK ONLY DISTILLED WATER

You will hear people say "Distilled water is dead water ... a fish cannot live in it." Of course a fish cannot live in freshly-distilled water for any length of time, because he needs the vegetation that grows in rivers, lakes, and seas.

Another erroneous notion about distilled water is that it "leaches the organic minerals out of the body." This is not only false but utterly absurd.

Distilled water helps to dissolve the terrible, morbid, putrid *toxic poisons that collect in civilized men's bodies.* It helps to eliminate these toxic poisons through the kidneys ... and it passes through the kidneys *without leaving inorganic pebbles and stones.*

Distilled water is the purest water that man can drink. Every liquid prescription that is compounded in any drug store the world over is prepared with distilled water. It is used in baby's formulas and for many hundreds of other purposes where absolutely pure water is essential.

Distilled water is soft water. If you wash your hair in distilled water you will discover how soft it is.

In thousands of homes there are water softeners for household use, because hard water is not good for the hands, the body, or for washing clothes. But please *do not drink the water from water softeners!* In my opinion, *it is not healthful drinking water,* because of its salt and chemical content.

At my home in Hollywood, California, distilled water is delivered in 5-gallon bottles for our household use, and I also have it in my office. Try distilled water exclusively for a year ... and you will never drink hard water again!

It's strange that some men will drink and eat anything put before them, but check very carefully the oil put in their car.

75

BALANCED BODY CHEMISTRY IMPORTANT

In this Heart Fitness Program I have been emphasizing the DON'TS because I consider these much more difficult to follow than the DO'S. Now, *what kind of food program shall we follow* for heart fitness, health and longer life?

Every time you plan a meal, check off *these five items* on the fingers of your hand to see if you are eating a *nutritionally well blanaced combination of foods:*

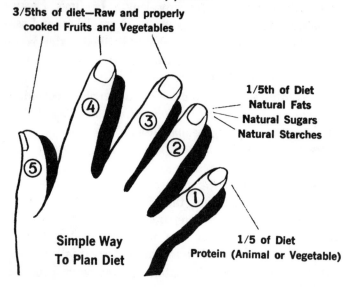

3/5ths of diet—Raw and properly cooked Fruits and Vegetables

1/5th of Diet Natural Fats Natural Sugars Natural Starches

Simple Way To Plan Diet

1/5 of Diet Protein (Animal or Vegetable)

Life is largely a matter of chemistry. —Wm. J. Mayo, M.D.

A recent cholesterol screening at the University of California, Davis, found that 61% of all men and 51% of all women exceeded the latest guidelines of the National Institutes of Health of less than 200 mg/dl of cholesterol.

Thirty years ago most medical schools taught that any cholesterol reading below 350 mg/dl was acceptable. The consensus today is that the level should be much lower—below 200 mg/dl for adults.

Healthy Fiber Habit: *Have 3 to 5 tablespoons of raw oat bran a day in juices, soups, herbal teas, pep drinks, cereals, muffins, etc. plus ample salads, fresh fruits, vegetables, legumes and 100% whole grains! Fiber helps reduce cholesterol and varicose veins. Fiber helps keep you regular and reduces hemorrhoids and is a natural body weight normalizer.*

PROTEIN—THE BUILDING BLOCKS OF THE BODY

Protein is one of the most important food elements, and *is essential for keeping the heart fit*. You must have protein for building every cell in the body. This fundamental Law of Nature rules every animal living on the face of the Earth.

Protein is YOU ... flesh, muscle, blood, heart, bones, skin, hair ... all the components of the body are essentially composed of protein. *You are literally "built" of protein.* This basic function of your body ... that of converting food into living tissue ... is one of the miracles of life itself. Your life processes ... the factors that help you resist disease ... are all composed of protein (amino-acids).

Every time you move a muscle, every time your heart beats, every time you breathe, you consume protein in the form of amino-acids. Without protein you would be a hopeless, helpless cripple. The link between protein and the body tissue is the amino-acids. When these enter the bloodstream they are carried to every part of the body, where they set to work repairing, rebuilding and maintaining body tissues, building up rich red blood, and "conditioning" the various bodily organs including the all-powerful heart.

PROTEIN FOODS are meat, fish, poultry, nuts, seeds (such as Sunflower, Sesame, Pumpkin), brewer's yeast, wheat-germ, soya beans, milk products, cereals and protein supplements.

MEATS AND DAIRY PRODUCTS

Beef, veal and lamb are naturally high in both visible and "invisible" fat and cholesterol. This is why we stress not to eat meat more than three to four times a week. (The average American man has bacon or ham for breakfast; a meat hamburger for lunch; steak or roast for dinner—which all adds up to a diet heavy in deadly cholesterol saturated fats.)

The more expensive meats—prime and choice grades have the highest content of fats, visible and "invisible," and are often force fattened. Buy the cheaper grades of meat—for these have less fat and are just as good.

Always trim off all visible fat before cooking. During the cooking, baking or broiling of the meat, the fat should drain off, by keeping the meat or roast on racks, so the meat will not soak in its own fat drippings.

Don't Eat Fried Foods. The frying pan is the cradle of indigestion, heart disease and death. The sputtering lumps of frying, sizzling fat are enemies of your heart and entire body.

Instead of fat-rich gravies, meats can be flavored with herbs, garlic, onions and tomatoes and mushrooms, etc. You can garnish meats attractively with a variety of raw vegetables such as: watercress, parsley, celery, carrots, radishes, green bell peppers, and cucumbers cut in various shapes and combinations. During the last five minutes of broiling meat, add a banana (sliced lengthwise) or a sliced apple to give a delicious flavor that is different.

Compared with meats, *fish is as a rule an excellent low fat protein*. I always try to get freshly caught fish, because it is the best both in taste and for health.

*Poultry—chicken and turkey—*are excellent sources of animal proteins and are also in the low fat and low cholesterol content, provided lean poultry is used. Guinea hen and squab are also comparatively low in fat content. But duck and goose are way too high in fat content, so it is best to enjoy the other lower fat-content poultry. Skins should be discarded and also giblets for they are high in fat content.

Eggs. If you must eat eggs, limit them to 3 or 4 per week. The yolk (yellow portion) of the egg contains a concentrated form of cholesterol fat.

Milk and its milk products should be forgotten on a low fat diet. We use no milk products and have not for years. We do not eat Yogurt because this also contains fat, unless it is specially made from non-fat milk. Cheeses are very high in butterfat content, and we advise limiting the amount of natural cheese eaten—or better still, not to eat cheese. We do not eat cheese, or even cottage cheese—for now they use strong chemicals to process it, so it is no longer a natural product.

The great thing in the world is not so much where we stand,
as in what direction we are moving.

CARBOHYDRATES—STARCHES AND SUGARS

Starches and sugars come under a single classification in the diet—Carbohydrates, which provide the principle source of food energy in the diet. Carbohydrates are needed as fuel for muscular work and physical activity. Excess sugars and starches that are not utilized as energy are changed by the body chemistry into fat and stored in the least active body parts.

Carbohydrates originate in plants as ... sugars formed by photosynthesis, then are formed into clusters as starches ... consumed by humans, and once more broken down by the body chemistry into the simple sugar, glucose, for use by the cells of the body. It is important that you eat only natural starches and sugars, and avoid those which have been depleted of vital elements (refined white flour, sugar, etc.).

NATURAL STARCHES AND SUGARS are found in all fresh fruits and vegetables,*raw sugar (not refined white sugar), honey, maple syrup, sorghum and molasses, whole grains (wheat, oats, rye, etc.) and whole grain flour, dried beans and peas, whole brown rice, potatoes. All natural foods, in fact, contain some carbohydrates.

HOW TO CHOOSE A FAT

Fat is also a source of energy in the diet ... in fact, it has more than twice the energy value of the same amount of carbohydrates or protein. As already pointed out in this Heart Fitness Program, a certain amount of fat is necessary and so is a certain amount of cholesterol. But let me remind you that your fat intake should be a preponderance of the unsaturated fats ... and the * saturated fats in meat, eggs, poultry and dairy products) should be kept to a minimum.

It is the saturated fats which overload our body with cholesterol. Cholesterol is a fatty substance produced daily by the liver for normal use in the body. But when we overload our bloodstream with cholesterol in our diet, it forms a waxy deposit on the walls of the arteries and blocks the flow of blood, as discussed earlier in this book.

* With severe heart problems best to remove from diet all simple sugars (raw sugar, honey, maple syrup and molasses) as well as fats, all oils, meats, eggs, dairy products and nuts until problem has corrected itself . . . usually within a matter of months, if diet, fasting and exercise are strict!

THE FUNCTION OF FAT IN THE BODY

Our nerves, muscles and organs must be "cushioned" by a normal amount of fat. If we did not have a certain amount of fat in our "gluteus maximus" (the buttocks), for example, we would never be able to sit down, because we would have to sit directly on our muscles and bones.

Those who wish to reduce should reduce the fat-content of their diet ... and those who wish to gain should increase it. But even if you are on a reducing diet, there should always be some fat in the menu because it plays an important role in the body chemistry. * pg 79

Stored in the body, fat provides a source of heat and energy, and the accumulation of a certain amount of fat around the vital organs (such as the kidneys) gives great protection against cold and injury.

Fat also has a function to perform in the body cells, for which special fats known as unsaturated fatty acids are needed in small amounts in the diet. Without these there is roughness or scaliness of the skin.

Fats have another all-important function ... they carry the fat-soluble Vitamins A, D, E and K in the body.

So, a certain amount of fat in the diet is essential to have a healthily functioning body. It is the kind of fat that is all-important! Unsaturated—YES! ... Saturated—NO!

THE COMMERCIAL CRIME AGAINST PEANUT BUTTER

Peanut butter is a fine food ... It is rich in vitamin B-complex ... the food for the nerves. It has been called the "Cinderella" of nutrition because it is one of the cheapest forms of high-nutritional food you can get. In "the good old days," before commercialism dominated our staple foods, the old-fashioned kind of peanut butter was simply ground-up peanuts with its own natural oil on the top. This peanut butter was natural, as peanut-oil that has not been "doctored" or hydrogenated is an unsaturated fat.

You are what you eat! What you eat today will be walking and talking tomorrow. — Paul C. Bragg

But on the shelves of the warm super-markets and grocery stores this natural peanut butter would take on oxygen and become rancid. This hurt the manufacturers of peanut butter where it hurt the most, and that was in their pocket-books! So the worst happened!

They took this wonderful, nutritious food and added saturated hydrogenated hard fat and even salt (which acts as a preservative). Then they ran extensive advertisements stating that this peanut butter is always fresh. Of course it is fresh, but it is kept fresh by the artificial process of hydrogenation! The producers of this peanut butter tell people it is easy to use and keeps longer, and that pleases the modern, unthinking housewife, who is easily brainwashed by the commercials.

Be sure to read labels! When you see the words "hydrogenated fat" . . . BEWARE! You would never find me consuming such products.

SAFFLOWER OIL HIGHLY RECOMMENDED

Nature has provided us with a wonderful unsaturated oil which can be used in preparing mayonnaise and salad dressings and for all cooking purposes. This oil was used by people in days gone by . . . but like many other wonderful foods, it was discarded with the "progress" of civilization. Now, thanks to Nutritional Science, it is once more coming back into its own.

The finest of all oils for human consumption are pure vegetable oils and safflower oil is one of the best. It is 72% poly-unsaturated and about 94% unsaturated fatty acids.

Cold-pressed corn oil is 55% poly-unsaturated and contains about 78% unsaturated fatty acids . . . cold-pressed soybean oil is 52% poly-unsaturated and contains about 70% unsaturated fatty acids with sesame oil and peanut oil running next.

Safflower oil also contains another important fatty acid—linoleic acid, which is absolutely essential to life itself. Safflower oil contains about 72% of this precious acid. Therefore,

---

Love is a fruit in all seasons and within reach of every hand - Mother Teresa

Safflower oil is my choice as the best oil to use in salads, cooking and baking.

(NOTE: The animal fat highest in unsaturated fatty acids is natural lard, and this contains only 5% to 11%. Most of the lard found in the supermarkets has been hydrogenated so that it will not become rancid ... thus reducing the unsaturated fatty acid content to an even lower percentage. Therefore, I do not recommend the use of commercial lard.)

THE PROTECTIVE FOODS—FRUITS AND VEGETABLES

Remember that I told you that three-fifths of your diet should be fruits and vegetables ... both raw in salads or desserts and properly cooked. These foods not only contribute vitamins and organic minerals to the diet ... but also add the bulk and moisture required for proper body functioning. They also help maintain the alkaline reserve of the body. They add variety, color, flavor and texture to the diet.

Vegetables are fat free and contain no cholesterol. The ideal way to get the full quota of vitamins and minerals from the vegetables is in their raw state, served in a fresh vegetable salad or as a garnish with your meat or roast or meat substitutes. When vegetables are cooked, some of the vitamins and minerals may be lost.

Vegetable juice freshly prepared is an ideal way to add vitamins and minerals to your daily diet. We enjoy carrot, celery and beet juice mixed together. You can also combine other vegetables that are equally delicious.

There are three Bragg Health Books which you will find helpful in planning your health-building diet. These are: **"Healthful Eating Without Confusion," "Bragg's Complete Health Gourmet Recipes For Vital Health,"** and our **"Vegetarian Gourmet Health Recipes** (no salt, no sugar). (Please see back pages for ordering.)

Nutrition directly affects growth, development, reproduction, well-being and the physical and mental condition of the individual. Health depends upon nutrition more than on any other single factor. —Dr. Wm. H. Sebrell, Jr.

THE IMPORTANCE OF LECITHIN

The liver, in addition to producing the body's normal cholesterol, also produces an important nutritional substance called lecithin. In my opinion, lecithin is one of God's greatest gifts to man. Lecithin mixes with the bile in the gall bladder, and is emptied along with the bile into the small intestine to help in the digestion of fats as these leave the stomach. Lecithin is a powerful homgenizing agent which breaks up the fat into tiny particles of uniform size and quality.

One of the great discoveries of modern Nutritional Science is the role of lecithin and linoleic acid (from safflower oil) in helping the body to dispose of fats. You can see that a deficiency of these two agents may cause nutritional coronary ailments.

The soybean is the richest source of lecithin. It is also found in all products which contain fat, such as the germ of the various grains (the part that sprouts). In appearance lecithin and wheat-germ are very much alike.

Commercial lecithin has a wide variety of uses. It is used in the lubrication of fine precision machines where the oil needs to be spread very thinly, and it is important in the confectionary and baking businesses for its natural homogenizing effect.

RACES WHO USE LECITHIN HAVE FEW HEART TROUBLES

In 1910 when I was one of the associate editors of Bernarr Macfadden's *Physical Culture Magazine,* he sent me on an expedition into Upper Manchuria in China. This is the original home of the soybean. For thousands of years the Chinese people have used the soybean as a food in many different ways. In fact, about 80% of their food has been soybean in one form or another.

Again, to my amazement I found many men and women like Zora Agha of Turkey, who were living unbelievably long lives. It was not unusual to find men and women from 125 to 135 years of age. Among these people heart attacks, strokes, paralysis, coronary thrombosis and degenerative diseases of the arteries were practically unknown. Eating the soybean in various forms meant that they got a large amount of lecithin in their diet which homogenized the fats ... and thus their level of blood-fat or blood cholesterol was always normal.

83

SOYBEAN POWDER FOR HEALTHY HEART AND NERVES

I have been recommending the use of soybeans and soybean powder to the health-conscious people of this country for more than 80 years.

Lecithin ... of which the soybean is the richest source ... not only is important in the digestion of fats. It is found in the nervous system and in every cell of the body. The functioning of the nervous system and the glands are greatly aided by the phospholipids, one of the most important constituents of lecithin.

It has been observed that nervous people and those who use their brains a great deal burn up more lecithin than people who are phlegmatic. Brain workers and nervous persons therefore need more of this valuable food-factor.

Nutritional Science teaches us that the nervous system requires both lecithin and Vitamin B-Complex every day.

THE VALUE OF RAW WHEAT-GERM AND VITAMIN E

Nature put into the grain of wheat the raw wheat-germ, which contains one of the most valuable vitamins, Vitamin E. And now it is coming to the aid of civilized man to help him regain the robust health he has lost through devitalized foods.

Dr. Cureton of the University of Illinois, recognized as the greatest living authority on internal and external physical fitness, highly recommends raw wheat-germ (little yellowish flakes), wheat germ oil and Vitamin E capsules as a great boost to athletes and others who desire to be in the highest form of physical fitness. Athletic coaches all over the world are following this advice for better performance from their athletes.

In my opinion, *raw wheat-germ, wheat-germ oil and Vitamin E should be included in the nutritional program of everyone* . . . not just athletes. I recommend capsule form, as in the gelatin capsule the oil never becomes rancid.

In the refinement of white flour the raw wheat-germ is removed. The millers know that the wheat-germ is an oily, fragile, natural capsule and will go rancid quickly. Commercial food demands a long shelf life. Mrs. Average Housewife

84

demands that everything she buys will never spoil. That is why so many American foods are refined and why more than 700 chemicals are used to preserve them!

Live, living, vital foods are perishable and spoil very quickly. So we have been ignorant, foolish and almost idiotic in allowing various foods to be tampered with and their vital and essential elements taken out of them. Some of this is done by so-called refinements, or in some cases sold in different forms. And we are buying and eating the depleted, devitalized material that remains. Nature will not stand for it...and our hearts and bodies suffer.

It is so wonderful that Nature will both build and repair if not interfered with. It is far better for us to understand and preserve the fine body balance for which Nature so abundantly supplies the material.

On mornings when I have natural whole grain cereal or Scotch Steel Oats, I slice a ripe banana over the cereal, add honey and then soy milk. I use a heaping teaspoon of pure soy bean powder mixed with 1/2 glass of cold distilled water in a jar & shake. It's delicious as well as healthful!

Even more delicious is the blended energy-drink which I have once a day. At our home it is called our favorite "Pep" Drink. Here is the recipe.

BRAGG "PEP" DRINK

Prepare in blender, add 1 ice cube if desired chilled:

Juice of 2-3 oranges (fresh) or unsweetened pineapple juice or 1 glass distilled water	1/2 tsp. Vitamin C powder
	1/3 tsp. pure pectin powder
	1-2 bananas, ripe
1 tbsp. raw wheat germ	1/3 tsp. flax seed oil
1 tsp. brewer's yeast	1 tsp. honey (optional)
1 tbsp. raw oat bran	1 tbsp. soy protein powder
1/2 tsp. psyllium husk powder	1 tsp. raw sunflower or
1 tbsp. lecithin granules	pumpkin seeds

Optional: 4 apricots (sun dried, unsulphured). Soak in jar overnight in distilled water or unsweetened pineapple juice. We soak enough to last for several days. Keep refrigerated. In summer you can add fresh fruit in season: peaches, strawberries, berries, apricots, etc., instead of the banana. In winter add apples, oranges, pears or persimmons or try sugar-free, frozen fruits.

Once you try this, you will understand why we call it our "Pep" Drink. It fills you with pep and energy and zest for living. It is really a meal in itself, and I usually take it for breakfast or lunch, or as a mid-afternoon pick-up.

THE IMPORTANCE OF CALCIUM IN HEART FITNESS

Most people associate calcium with the teeth and bones, which is correct, as a deficiency of this important mineral will bring on a serious condition of the bones and the teeth. Calcium is also very important for the nerves of the body, and many people suffer from leg cramps due to a calcium deficiency.

And calcium plays a very important role in the functioning of the human heart. Calcium is a natural constituent of material that causes the blood to clot. If we did not have calcium in our bloodstream we could prick a finger with a needle and bleed to death.

Every few minutes the heart is bathed by the calcium of the body chemistry. It is important to the very life of the heart's activity. Being the most powerful muscle in the entire body, the heart requires adequate calcium for its normal functioning.

Now consider the shocking condition that *85% of the American people are deficient in calcium!*

MILK—A CARRIER OF SATURATED FATS

Nearly everyone has the idea that if he drinks milk, the problem of calcium deficiency will be solved. This is not completely true. In the first place, practically all the milk in the United States is *pasteurized*, which reduces the availability of *the milk's calcium*.

Dr. Harold D. Lynch, author, researcher and physician of Evansville, Indiana, said recently that the "almost fanatic use of milk as a beverage has added more complications than benefits to child nutrition." He stated that *milk may often be a primary cause of poor nutrition in children.*

When you realize that each body cell is a small factory, needing constant recharging through the food you eat, you'll begin to really think about diet.
—Dr. J.D. Nolan

To be properly utilized in the body chemistry calcium must have a proportionate amount of phosphorus and Vitamins A and D, which increase the ability of the body to absorb calcium.

Whole milk, as we have discovered, is a carrier of large amounts of saturated fat (cholesterol). When consumed in excessive amounts it may lead to arterosclerosis. In my opinion food for calves and babies should not be used by adults . . . that is, if they wish to maintain a healthy heart!

There are several very fine sources of calcium other than milk. I believe that raw bonemeal is one of the best, as well as eggshell calcium, oyster shell calcium and bone marrow calcium. Then there is the calcium which is found in corn and in wheat. In fact, as Dr. Lynch pointed out, all natural foods contain appreciable amounts of calcium.

THE TRUTH ABOUT SALT

Would you use sodium, a caustic alkali, to season your food? Or chlorine, a poisonous gas? "Ridiculous questions," you say. "Nobody would be foolhardy enough to do that."

Of course not. But the shocking truth is that most people do so . . . because they don't know that these powerful chemicals constitute the inorganic crystaline compound—salt.

For centuries, the expression "salt of the earth" has been used as a catch-all phrase to designate something good and essential. Nothing could be more erroneous. For that harmless product that you shake into your food every day may actually bury you. Consider these startling facts:

1. *SALT IS NOT A FOOD!* There is no more justification for its culinary use than there is for potassium chloride, calcium chloride, barium chloride, or any other harmful chemical to season food.

2. *Salt cannot be digested, assimilated, or utilized by the body.* Salt has no nutritional value! SALT HAS NO VITAMINS! NO ORGANIC MINERALS! NO NUTRIENTS OF ANY KIND! Instead, it is positively harmful and may bring

on troubles in the kidneys, bladder, heart, arteries, veins, and blood vessels. Salt may waterlog the tissues, causing a dropsical condition.

3. *Salt may act as a heart poison.* It also increases the irritability of the nervous system.

4. *Salt acts to rob calcium from the body* and attacks the mucous lining throughout the entire gastrointestional tract.

WHAT SALT DOES TO YOUR BLOOD PRESSURE

What causes high blood pressure? Medical Science knows of many causes: tension, strains, stress, toxic substance such as cigarets and gasoline fumes, food additives, insecticide sprays, the side effects of drugs, and industralization are suspect. What can you do to protect yourself from these causative agents? It is well to exclude as many of these harmful agents from your environment as possible!

However, there is one cause of high blood pressure which can be remedied. *Sodium chloride (common table salt) is the major cause of high blood pressure.*

Up to now, we have been talking about causing high blood pressure in the "normal" person. But how about the effects of salt on those millions suffering from our country's most prevalent ailment, OVERWEIGHT. Here is a sensitive area for research, because overweight is known to be frequently accompanied by high blood pressure. Is there a link between the overweight individual's high blood pressure and his salt intake? Top medical researchers say, "Yes."

THE MYTH OF THE "SALT LICK"

Is a low-salt diet a deficient diet? Don't we need plenty of salt in our diets to keep us in top physical condition? This is a popular notion ... but is it true? People will tell you that animals will travel for miles to visit the so-called "salt licks." I investigated the salt-licks where wild forest animals congregated from miles around to lick the soil. Although all of these sites were known as "salt licks" the one chemical property they all had in common was *complete absence of sodium chloride (common salt)*. There was absolutely NO organic or inorganic sodium at the salt licks. *But they had an abundance of many organic minerals* and nutrients which the animals craved.

SALT IS NOT ESSENTIAL TO LIFE

It is frequently claimed that salt is essential for the support of life. However, there is no information available to substantiate this viewpoint. The truth is that entire races (primitive peoples) use absolutely no salt today and have not used it throughout their entire history. If salt were essential to life, these races would have become extinct long ago. The fact that they are not only alive but have far better health than other races, would seem to indicate that the supposed "necessity" of salt is a commercially-inspired invention or merely the product of the imagination.

SALT IS NOT NECESSARY TO COMBAT HEAT

There has been a great deal of propaganda in recent years about using salt in hot weather. The claim is made that the body loses much salt in perspiration and that this loss must be compensated for by consuming additional amounts of salt —otherwise, supposedly great weakness and inability to continue normal activities will result. Hence factory workers are advised to take salt tablets in hot weather. I have seen many factory workers take these salt tablets and I have also seen many of them become quite ill afterward. The most toxic reactions frequently follow the use of salt tablets. Vomiting and indigestion appear to be the most common after effects, and, so far as enabling one to stand the heat better is concerned, it is not agreed that salt tablets do this.

I have repudiated this "salt for hot weather" superstition many times. I have a home on the great colorful Colorado Desert of California, and from the first of June until the first of October we have continuous, blazing heat of from 110° to sometimes 130° ... but *I never* use salt, and I issue a standing challenge that I can out-do any man alive in an endurance test even in this desert heat. I will let him use all the salt tablets he desires and I will use absolutely no salt, and I know from experience in the desert that I will defeat him in any test of endurance.

In my expeditions over the world I have met many *primitive tribes* in the tropics that *use no salt*, and they are not bothered by the heat, whereas salt-eating white people invariably complain of hot weather. This seems to indicate that some commercial motive lies behind the "eat more salt in hot weather" campaign.

WHAT SALT DOES TO YOUR STOMACH

An important objection to salt is the fact that it *interferes with* the *normal digestion of food*. Pepsin, an enzyme found in the hydrochloric acid of the stomach, is essential for the digestion of proteins. When salt is used, only 50% as much pepsin is secreted as would otherwise be the case. Obviously, under such conditions, digestion of protein foods is incomplete or too slow. The result is excessive putrefaction of protein and, in some instances, gas and digestive distress.

THE SALT HABIT IS A DEADLY HABIT—BREAK IT!

People undoubtedly would not add inorganic salt to their food if they were never taught to do so in the first place. *The taste for salt is an acquired one.* When salt is eliminated from the diet for a short time, the craving for it ceases. It is only during the first few weeks after table salt is discontinued that it is really missed ... after that, abstinence is of little difficulty. In fact, many of my health students ... who have broken the deadly salt habit ... write me that NOW they cannot stand salted foods! When someone serves them salted food, it gives them an abnormal thirst for liquids.

Many outstanding heart specialists heartily endorse a NO SALT DIET. To satisfy the acquired craving for salt in food, there are excellent salt substitutes that are sodium free. In the Bragg home we use powdered sea kelp, herb and vegetable seasonings.

90

SEA KELP—AN EXCELLENT SALT SUBSTITUTE

In my opinion, sea kelp is the ideal salt substitute. It gives all food—salads, vegetables, meats, fish, etc.—a tangy taste. Granular sea kelp may be purchased at any Health Food Store.

There are also many herbs with which you may flavor your food as a substitute for ordinary salt. Pure garlic powder, for example, makes an excellent seasoner. Lemon juice is particularly good for seasoning meat and fish.

Take a lesson from famous French chefs! The marvelous flavor of world-renowned French dishes is achieved by the skillful use of onions, garlic, mushrooms and herbs ... not with salt! French cooking is called "rich"—but it is a richness of taste, not of content. The best French chefs use very little fat and very little salt—and some use no salt at all!

YOUR TASTE BUDS WILL TELL YOU

After you give up salt you will appreciate the natural flavor of foods. I was born and reared in the South where salt was used plentifully in the seasoning of nearly all foods. My 260 taste buds were conditioned to the heavy taste of salt.

At the age of 16 I was a victim of T.B. and was placed in a "NATURE SANATORIUM" in Switzerland. Dr. Rollier, who operated this sanatorium was against salt in the diet. At first my taste buds rebelled. But no salt was permitted ... so I re-educated my taste buds to a saltless diet. Any bad habit is difficult to overcome at first, and the salt habit surely had me in its clutches. But once my taste buds learned the difference, for the first time in my life I started to taste and enjoy the real, natural flavors of food.

Now I cannot stand to eat salted foods of any kind. That is why it is difficult for me to eat out in a restaurant, because all food in commercial establishments is usually heavily salted. But I have solved that problem, too. When I go into a restaurant, I simply say, "Do not salt my food." I order a la carte my special salad of mixed fresh vegetables and my other dishes prepared to my instructions—NO SALT!

Some health-minded people use *sea salt* rather than *common salt*. There is absolutely no difference between these two salts. They are *both inorganic* and *both loaded with deadly sodium-chloride*.

After you have discarded salt from your diet, your 260 taste buds will tell you the difference. They will become very keen and sensitive and will reject salty foods. You will really begin to enjoy tasting all the natural flavors of foods.

OUR NATURAL FOODS CONTAIN PLENTY OF ORGANIC SODIUM

Organic sodium is one of the 16 minerals that are *necessary to have perfect mineral balance* in the human body. Sodium is the most plentiful organic mineral found in all fruits and vegetables, especially *beets and celery*. You may be assured that by eating a balanced diet with a wide variety of natural foods you will have plenty of organic sodium.

AGAIN LET ME WARN YOU—If you want a powerful, long lasting heart, *put down that salt shaker and never pick it up again!*

DON'T OVER-EAT!

Second after second, minute after minute, hour after hour, day after day, our faithful, loyal heart is working to keep us alive. In our waking hours as well as our sleeping time, our heart takes only a sixth of a second to rest between beats.

The hardest work the heart has to do is right after the individual has eaten. The bigger the meal, the more work it has to do in pumping vast quantities of blood into the digestive tract.

Over-eating puts more strain on the heart than any other one thing. Many people load up on a ten-course dinner ... and afterward suffer a heart attack. Over-eating is a vicious habit that can only lead to serious consequences.

You should always get up from the table feeling that you could eat a little more.

Don't injure your system by over-feeding it.

92

LIGHT EATERS LIVE LONGER

In all the scientific tests made on controlled animal feeding, it has been conclusively proved that light eaters live longer and retain the prime of life longer. In my own research in interviewing men and women who remained vigorous at ages well over 100 years, all ate sparingly. They never over-ate ... and their diets were well balanced natural foods.

Eat slowly! Make it a principle of your Nutrition Program always to *eat slowly* and *chew your food thoroughly*. Never eat in a hurry. Food bolted into the stomach can cause much trouble and overwork the heart. It can produce gas pressure on the heart ... and many a heart attack has resulted from this very cause. If you do not have sufficient time to eat correctly, skip that meal! Occasionally skipping meals is a good habit to form.

Most eating habits are formed early in life and set a pattern for future eating. To live long, to feel youthful, and to have a powerful heart, you must be able to avoid or get rid of bad habits and condition yourself to healthy eating habits.

FASTING—THE HEART-RESTER

If you are vitally interested in having a strong heart, you must get into the habit of skipping one or two meals or even fasting for a whole day at a time. What a wonderful rest the hardworking heart receives when you take a day or two of fasting—complete abstinence from all food! Just drink quantities of cool distilled water . . . and if you feel you need something warm, have a cup of herb tea, such as mint, alfalfa, anise seed, etc., and you may add ½ teaspoon of honey if desired. But partake of no juices or food during a fast.

THE STORY OF SUCCESSFUL FASTING

In my files I have many interesting letters from health students all over the world, who have done remarkable things with fasting. At 55 years of age one of these students, had a serious heart attack. She was in bed flat on her back for eight weeks. When she finally got up she was a pitiful sight—pale, haggard and weak. She was thoroughly discouraged, as she was told that she did not have long to live.

Then she got hold of the Bragg book *THE MIRACLE OF FASTING* and started to fast one day each week. After a few months she fasted 3 or 4 days each month. Then she went on a 7-day complete fast. Great changes of a beneficial nature took place in her body from her fasting and correct eating program.

(NOTE: The Bragg Book *THE MIRACLE OF FASTING* is a complete and instructive program on the Science of Fasting. See inside back page of this book for details.)

BANISH ALL YOUR FEARS ABOUT FASTING

The average person has a preconceived notion that if he skips a few meals or fasts for a few days, dangerous things will happen to his body. Nothing is farther from the truth! I have fasted for as many as 30 days straight . . . and have been stronger on the 30th day than when I started. CAUTION: I do not advise my students to go on long fasts unless they are supervised. There are Health Spas that will supervise fasts in many parts of the world.

Nothing will give the body energy and vitality and strengthen the digestive system and the heart more than fasting. Forget your fears! Fasting cleanses the internal "house" of your body. Try a short fast and demonstrate to yourself what fasting can and will do for you.

Let me pass on my regular fasting program to you. On Mondays I eat my usual meals . . . but from Monday night to Tuesday dinner I eat nothing. During this time I drink only distilled water. I give my digestive and elimination system a complete rest. I skip breakfast and lunch, then eat my dinner Tuesday evening. This takes a great load off my hardworking heart as well as my digestive system.

Several times each year I take a longer "super" fast. I go on a complete distilled water fast for an entire week. This means no vegetable juices or fresh fruit. It is a complete fast. And it works wonders in keeping me fit!

94

MY SYSTEM OF CLEANSING THE GREAT PUMP
AND PIPES OF THE BODY

If our "pipes" and great "pump" are clogged and corroded with debris and poisons, we cannot be physically fit. Therefore, I think it is necessary from time to time to give the "pipes" and the "pump" of the body a thorough cleansing. This cleansing should be done for at least 1 to 3 days ... even one day will have beneficial effects. It will vibrate and shake the tissues, thereby stimulating the circulation and getting rid of foreign matter that has been stored in the heart and blood vessels.

You should carry out this cleansing program at least one day a month ... and the person who has fortitude enough to do it for 3 days straight will be amazed at the results. If during this cleansing program you feel any reactions, such as headaches, excessive gas or feelings of weakness, just remember it is what we call a "healing crisis" and those symptoms will pass away when the poisons pass out through the elimination system.

FLUSHING THE POISONS FROM THE "PIPES"

On this Pump-and-Pipe Cleansing Program at least one-half gallon of distilled water should be consumed daily during the waking hours. *No other water can act as a substitute for distilled water.* The night before you start this Cleansing Program take one quart of distilled water and add to it 1 whole carrot cut into pieces, 3 stalks of celery (leaves and all) also cut, 1 handful of parsley chopped, and 1 beet cut up fine. *Soak this mixture overnight.* After it has soaked 10 hours or more, strain the distilled water and discard the vegetables. Use this quart of water, in which the vegetables have been soaked, as your drinking water only between your meals during the first day.

On arising drink one glass of fruit juice, eat an apple, 2 medium-sized carrots and some dried figs or dates.

Many people aim to do right, but are just poor shots.

At 10:00 A.M. eat some kind of fresh fruit (oranges, grapefruit, bananas, apples, pears, grapes) and drink a cup of herb tea or vegetable broth. If you customarily take a dietary supplement, do so at this time.

At 12:00 Noon have a luncheon of a tossed green salad of grated cabbage with carrots and beets, chopped green onion, celery, sweet bellpepper, parsley, raw spinach, watercress, tomato and a clove of garlic finely chopped ... with a dressing made of 2 tablespoonsful of safflower, olive or soy oil to 1 tablespoonful of lemon juice; some kind of 5% cooked vegetables (low in sugar) such as stringbeans, squash or any greens; a cup of hot distilled water to which a protein concentrate (liquid aminos) may be added, or a vegetable (meatless) broth.

At 3:00 P.M. eat a piece of fresh fruit or dried fruits such as dates, figs, prunes, apple, grapes, banana, etc.

At 6:00 P.M. your supper consists of a tossed green salad made with a wide variety of raw vegetables as suggested for lunch; a dish of lightly steamed greens (mustard greens, turnip greens, beet tops, spinach, etc.) cooked with a whole onion, chopped, a clove of garlic and 2 tablespoonsful of safflower or soy oil. You may also take regular dietary supplements at this time.

During the day be sure that you drink the quart of distilled water in which you soaked the vegetables overnight, as this helps accelerate the cleansing within the heart and circulatory system.

SOUND SLEEP IS NECESSARY TO BUILD A STRONG HEART

Primitive men and women arise at daybreak and the early hours of their days are spent in physical activity. About mid-day they eat their largest meal; then immediately they lie down and rest, taking a good nap or sleep. (Just as babies and young children do today.) In an hour or so they wake up refreshed—ready for the other half of the day. Then they are active again until sundown, and at sundown they go to sleep again. So primitive man is awake about 12 hours and asleep about 12 hours.

96

Modern, civilized man gets up and drives himself all day long at high-pressure. His day is filled with stresses, strains, worries and cares. A daily nap or "siesta" (as the Spanish people call it) is unknown in his daily routine. All day long he takes stimulants to keep himself going ... coffee, tea, alcohol, cigarets, excessive amounts of sugar, candy, ice-cream ... everything to keep his poor body up to "concert pitch."

He lives in a modern age and at night he has brilliant lights to keep him awake. His amusements and entertainments all begin at night. The night clubs turn on their brightest lights, moving pictures lure him in to see exciting and fabulous stories on the screen ... television, the radio, parties ... everything seems to be geared to stimulate him. Instead of going to bed he drives himself, chasing the elusive thing called "happiness."

When he gets sleepy he can take a pill that can keep him awake, or he can drink some strong coffee or poisonous alcohol. He is constantly tightening his nervous system—all of which has a disastrous effect on the heart.

Modern man's nerves are so jangled and frazzled that when he goes to bed it is often impossible for him to sleep. As a result, *Americans consume tons of sleeping pills and tranquilizers* to try to calm their exhausted nervous systems.

Modern man goes 'round and 'round in a squirrel cage of his own making! Is it any wonder that ... in addition to the *soaring rate of heart disease in the United States* ... we have more people in *mental institutions than ever before in the history of the world?* A half-million American men and women are committed to mental institutions every year. These are now so overcrowded that they present one of our great problems of today.

You cannot have a strong heart, a sound mind and a healthy nervous system if you do not get enough good, sound, restful sleep.

Money will buy a bed, but not sleep; books, but not brains; food, but not appetite; finery, but not beauty; a house, but not a home; medicine, but not health; luxuries, but not culture; amusements, but not happiness; religion, but not salvation.

SLEEP IS ESSENTIAL NOT ONLY TO HEALTH— BUT TO LIFE ITSELF

Sleep is one of the first essentials in building and maintaining a strong, vital heart.

Sleep is more necessary than food. One can fast for many days, or many weeks if necessary, without any serious disadvantage if he is well-nourished before beginning the fast and has a satisfactory food-supply after its conclusion; but no one can 'fast' from sleep for more than a few days at a time without experiencing ill-effects.

One can scarcely endure an entire week of absolute sleeplessness. In early English history condemned criminals were put to death by being deprived of sleep, and the same method has been employed in China. Enforced sleeplessness, in fact, has been used as a form of torture by the Chinese—being more feared than any other. The men subjected to this frightful ordeal always die raving maniacs . . . These facts illustrate only too well the imperative necessity for sleep!

HOW MUCH SLEEP DO WE NEED?

How much sleep do we need? This is a question which cannot be answered arbitrarily as applying in all cases. Individuals differ. Without doubt, some persons require more sleep than others.

No definite rule can be laid down as to the amount of sleep required by different individuals. Those possessing the greatest amount of vitality and the strongest organisms require less sleep than those of limited vitality and weak functional powers. Those possessing a strong functional system and great vitality are able to build up energy during sleep and recuperate from exertions of the preceding day more rapidly than those less favored in this respect. In other words, a strong man can be quickly rested. His system can more rapidly repair the wear and tear of his daily work than that of a weak man.

Without doubt, *most people need from 7 to 8 hours sleep daily* . . . some of them need more, particularly women and children, who in many cases require 9 to 10 hours sleep or even more. I would say, as a general statement, that 8 hours of sleep per day is absolutely necessary for a strong heart, and 1 to 2 hours of this sleep should be obtained before midnight. One hour's sleep before midnight is worth three hours of sleep after midnight.

RULES FOR RESTFUL SLEEP

You should *sleep with your head to the north*, so that you will be in direct contact with the Earth's vibrations. You should sleep on an *outside porch* or in a room with *cross-ventilation*. When weather permits you should sleep completely nude, otherwise in *non-constricting night garments*. You should sleep without a pillow ... but if you do require one, sleep on a soft, baby pillow so that the head is not too high and the heart won't have to pump the blood so high against gravity.

For restful sleep you must take command of your lazy body, which often wants to fall asleep just any old way. Sleeping in a cramped position, or on too soft a mattress, or in such a way that the circulation is blocked ... is not restful sleep.

One should sleep on a firm mattress, or place a board under a soft one. This allows the muscles to stretch in natural relaxation, and relieves pressure on vital organs.

When on my world lectures tours, I often have to move the mattress onto the floor, for it be more firm. Seems some of the world's top hotels put their money into showy lobbies, and not into firm mattresses. Also in many homes which I visit, I often find sagging, old mattresses—but new cars in the garage.

At my Desert home I recently had a new bed platform made. It is just a flat piece of board with four legs on castors and upon this goes the firm mattress. It might take you a few nights to be accustomed to being stretched out flat—but your body will thank you.

I travel all over the world in trains, planes, ships, buses, and automobiles ... and I use *soft foam ear plugs* to shut out unnecessary sounds and noises. I feel it is absolutely necessary that we should *sleep in a place that is quiet!* Even though we often do fall asleep when there is noise all about us, the vibratory action of the noises has a direct effect on the heart, circulation and nervous system.

I believe that individuals should *sleep alone*. Two people sleeping in one bed is not healthy, because there are always toxins being released from the body and these toxins can be absorbed. Then there is also the noise of a person who breathes too deeply, snores, or is restless ... all of which interferes with the other person's sleep. It has been proved by scientific research that a person gets a better night's rest and stores up more vitality when he sleeps alone.

Married couples will wake up more refreshed sleeping next to each other—but each in his/her own twin bed. If this is not acceptable, then a king size bed is certainly preferable to the usual small double bed.

TAKE A DAILY "SIESTA"

If you *wish* to build a *strong heart* and a *strong nervous system*, take a mid-day nap. Getting an hour's rest (or whatever amount of time you can spare) in the middle of the day is just like beginning two days in one, because when you wake up after your mid-day nap or "siesta" you have stored up a terrific reserve of nervous energy. I think the people of Mexico, South America, Spain, France and Italy have the right idea when they make it a Federal law to close down every business from noon to 2 P.M. Sleep and rest are important when building a powerful body and heart!

A FRANK TALK TO HEART SUFFERERS

Do not be discouraged because you have an ailing or damaged heart. By following a program of clean, natural living you will probably live out your life span. Your wonderful body possesses great recuperative powers which, if fully utilized, are of tremendous help even in the most serious cases of heart trouble.

Think of yourself as a "battery"—you discharge energy and you must recharge yourself with proper food, rest and constructive emotions.

100

**Here are the points for you to remember in
Your Own Special Heart Fitness Program:**

- Absolutely no smoking or drinking.
- Plenty of sleep and relaxation.
- Don't let anybody or anything put undue pressures on you. Worry, stress, tension and strain do not cause heart attack—but they do not help to heal it, either.
- Eat simple, natural foods. Above all—don't over eat!
- Eat slowly and chew your food thoroughly. Chewing is the first process in digestion.
- Get plenty of regular exercise. Although complete rest may be necessary during the acute stage of your heart attack or when the heart is very weak ... as soon as this stage is past you will find properly regulated exercise a great help in rebuilding and revitalizing the heart and circulation.
- Don't get into emotional arguments. These waste your precious nervous energy. Walk away from unpleasant people or situations.
- Get the Happiness Habit. A cheerful, happy disposition can do much to prolong life.
- Keep away from all artificial stimulants—coffee, tea, cola drinks, alcohol. Don't let anyone tell you that alcohol will help your heart—that is a deadly lie.
- Walk! Breathe deeply ... and walk, walk, walk!
- A vegetarian diet is the best — if meat is desired, eat only lean, rare meat ... trim every bit of fat from it. Limit your intake of meat to 2 or 3 times per week. Eat unsaturated vegetarian proteins instead ... such as soybeans, tofu, sunflower seeds, sesame seeds, pumpkin seeds, and nuts such as almonds, pecans, peanuts, brazil, hazel, walnut and pine nuts.
- Absolutely NO SALT!
- No dairy products of any kind. Milk and cheese are high in saturated fats.
- If you must have eggs, eat only 2 or 3 weekly.
- Fruits and vegetables ... both raw and properly cooked ... should form at least 50 percent of your diet.
- Don't use concentrated chemical sugar substitute sweetners. They are made from harmful chemicals.
- Use honey, and use it sparingly.

- Fast during one 24-hour period every week. This will give your heart and other vital organs a physiological rest ... and help reduce the deadly cholesterol in your arteries.
- Remember—low-fat diet and exercise will help you keep your cholesterol level down to normal.

MY PERSONAL OPINION OF HEART TRANSPLANTS

When the first heart transplants were announced the newspapers reported every detail. This was the kind of news that the average civilized person wanted to hear. If your heart goes bad ... all you have to do is to have another one put in its place. Sounds wonderful! Why take care of your original heart when you can get a new one if the old one falls apart?

Human nature always wants the easy way out.

The first experiments with heart transplants were, of course, done with animals. The medical researchers reasoned that if heart transplants would work on animals, they would work on humans. *Dr. Barnard of Africa* performed heart transplants on 50 dogs ... none of them lived.

The actual operation is a rather uncomplicated procedure. If success were judged by the patient's condition during the first 24 hours only, there would undoubtedly be a very low mortality rate. But after two days the problem—which at this stage of our knowledge is unsurmountable—begins to develop. It is precisely the same problem that could not be solved in the animal experiments.

The body survives only because it fights off invasion of foreign substances such as toxic poisons, bacteria and viruses. The same mechanism leads it to attack the transplanted heart and destroy it. This same difficulty is still apparent in kidney transplants, which today have a survival rate of only about 5%.

The big problem in heart and kidney transplants is rejection. The human body will have absolutely nothing to do with a foreign substance. No matter how healthy the new heart or kidney may be, it is not a natural part of the body into which it is being put. To date medical science has found nothing with which to overcome this rejection of a new organ by the body. And in my opinion they never will.

I wish I were able to say that I believe it will work ... but the facts of Nature are almost completely against it. To me, the human heart transplant seems at present to be merely a sophisticated effort to carry on human experimentation.

Today many facts are available to show how heart disease can be avoided. That is the reason this Heart Fitness Program is written. It is to help prevent heart conditions. I have NO CURE FOR HEART DISEASE. I am not in the curing business. I agree thoroughly with the American Heart Association that through regular daily exercise and a scientifically balanced diet, a healthy heart can be assured.

BUILD A HEALTHY HEART FOR YOURSELF

Personally, I do not believe in heart transplants. I believe that the first thing you should do is to live life so that you will not damage your heart. In this Heart Fitness Program I have told you in detail about the vicious enemies of the heart. Know your enemies and keep away from them!

If you have lived a haphazard life and have damaged your heart I believe that you can make a comeback and build a healthy heart for yourself. Remember the body is self-healing and self-repairing ... and given the chance it will do its best to rebuild a vigorous heart for you. But you must work with Nature—not against it.

General public knowledge of the heart is crammed with fallacies as well as facts. Let's consider some of these misconceptions.

MUST THE HEART PATIENT WITH CORONARY TROUBLES REST ALL THE TIME?

No! The belief that a "coronary" always means the end of useful life is widespread—and wrong. Most coronary occlusions (heart attacks) involve only a small branch of the "coronary tree" system of blood vessels. The blocked artery may be bypassed by the collateral channels which lie unused in the heart tissues awaiting just this eventuality. The new circulatory route may be so efficient that, after recovery, the patient may have no disability at all or else only on extreme exertion.

Certainly in the acute phase of the attack, the process of healing is assisted if the body is rested. The degree and duration of inactivity should be decided by your own doctor.

Once healing is complete, however, further rest rarely achieves anything of value. To the contrary, it is likely to increase disability by adding the ill effects of physical unfitness and lack of self-confidence.

IS EXERTION HARMFUL AFTER A HEART ATTACK?

This is a variation of the same theme as the need for rest . . . and is usually just as wrong.

The heart has enormous reserves of power which are seldom, if ever, used in ordinary living. It is this reserve which enables individuals to perform apparently superhuman feats in times of crisis or emergency. Athletes call upon this reserve —the runner who covers a mile in less than four minutes, for example, or the 50-mile endurance swimmer.

Even after many heart attacks, the reserve power of the heart is not greatly decreased and is available for use. It should not be abused, of course. Generally, the heart patient who over-exerts himself will develop warning symptoms—a special kind of chest pain and breathlessness. This is Nature's way of telling him to slow down. Similar symptoms, however, may be the result of physical unfitness, unusual stress or tension, emotional upsets and fatigue.

The thing I want you to remember is that *your body is always undergoing change.* You are not the person this minute that you were a minute ago. The body is always in ceaseless change, for better or worse. Every minute of your life old cells are being sluffed off and new ones are taking their places.

The question you must ask yourself is: "What kind of new body cells am I making? Are these body cells being built with healthy food or unhealthy food?"

104

If you drink alcohol, coffee, tea, cola drinks, eat refined white bread and refined sugar, overload on salt and salted foods and rich, fatty foods...you are going to make weak body cells that will decay and cause you plenty of trouble. On the other hand, if you follow the instructions given in this Heart Fitness Program, you are going to help your body rebuild a stronger heart and a stronger body. It's all in your hands. I can only help you to help yourself.

If you have had a heart condition, start NOW ... systematically and efficiently ... to build a fit heart for the old. Never think that "a bad ticker" necessarily means farewell to activity which can be a major part of the enjoyment of life.

Face your problem and start changing your bad habits of living into good habits. This is a mental and a physical process. Your mind must control your body. Never let the body be in command. That is the duty of the mind and it must have absolute obedience to its will. The whole person is at his best when mind and body work as a team. Then you have health supreme.

DR. JOHN HARVEY KELLOGG'S FAMOUS VEGETARIAN DIET FOR HEART SUFFERERS

Dr. John Harvey Kellogg was the founder and for many years the *director of the great Battle Creek Sanitarium at Battle Creek, Michigan.* Sick people from all over the world— even Royalty—came to be under his personal care.

I was fortunate to be associated with this great doctor for several years at Battle Creek, and to study his methods.

As soon as a heart attack victim was brought to the Sanitarium, Dr. Kellogg would put him on a strict vegetarian diet, with the advice that this should be a lifetime diet. It was a strict, exclusively vegetarian regime, consisting of fruit, vegetables, seeds and nuts. No meat, no fish, no eggs, no dairy products, no coffee, no alcohol, no salt.

Use your will power and better judgement to select and eat only the foods which are best for you, regardless of the ridicule or gibes of your friends or acquaintances. —Dr. Richard T. Field

Here are a few of Dr. Kellogg's Menus:

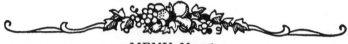

MENU No. 1
Breakfast

Natural Sun-Dried Apricots*
topped with Raw Wheat Germ and
Sliced Banana or Orange (if desired)
*soak in jar overnight in distilled water
or unsweetened pineapple juice
Or
you may substitute any morning the
Bragg Health Pep Drink on page 85 for a delicious
energy breakfast...remember you must earn your
breakfast with some form of exercise first.

Lunch
Raw Vegetable Combination Salad
consisting of
Grated Raw Beet, Carrot, Cabbage, Zucchini and Parsley*
over top spread chopped Tomato and Green Onions
Salad Dressing
made of
Fresh Lemon or Orange and Olive Oil* *
with a trace of Honey
1/3 Cup of Sunflower or Pumpkin Seeds
(rich in Protein and Natural Oil)
Raw Apple
*sprouts, alfalfa, mung, and sunflowers are delicious
added to all salads
**Also try Flaxseed or Jojoba oil

Dinner
Tossed Green-Leaf Salad
with
Raw Chopped Spinach, Kale, Cucumber,
Celery, Parsley, and Tomato
Lemon or Orange and Olive Oil Dressing
Protein – Vegetable
Fresh Fruit

106

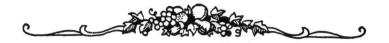

MENU No. 2

Breakfast
Apple Sauce*
Steel Cut Oats—hot cereal**
served with Natural Molasses,
honey or maple syrup
Whole Wheat Toast

*Make your own Apple Sauce, if desired add Honey
**Top and serve with Sliced Ripe Banana or other Fruit

Lunch

Raw Vegetable Combination Salad
(Same as 1st Day)
Vegetable Soup with Natural Barley, and Lentils
Whole Rye Toast or Oat Bran—Raisin Muffin

Dinner
Cabbage & Carrot Cole Slaw with Spring Onions

Baked Potato (or) Brown Rice
(Eat potato skin)
Baked or Steamed Carrots

Fresh Fruit
(or)
Avocado and Tomato Salad
Asparagus   Broccoli
Raw Nuts of any kind
Fresh Fruit

*Habits of rapid eating are most harmful, and must be overcome.
Quietness and Cheerfulness at meals is most essential for health.
– Oliver Wendell Holmes*

*You are a Miracle - Self-Healing, Self-Repairing — Please become aware of
"YOU" and be thankful for all your many blessings that take place daily!*

*Healthy Habit: Substitute raw honey or unsulfured blackstrap molasses instead
of sugar - use sparingly 1/3 amount as both are sweeter.*

Dr. Kellogg believed that the strict vegetarian diet was the only one which a heart sufferer should eat, because this was a diet free of cholesterol. It was also a salt-free diet. As beverages, the only drinks allowed were herb teas, fresh fruit and vegetable juices and distilled water.

Dr. Kellogg told me that serious heart cases who had come to him had lived as many as 50 years after the heart damage on this strict vegetarian diet.

Dr. Kellogg himself lived and practiced until he was well up into his nineties. He adhered strictly to a lacto-vegetarian diet, adding a small amount of natural cheese several days a week and 3 eggs weekly to the otherwise completely vegetarian diet which he advocated for his heart patients. At age 92 he was still performing delicate operations at his Sanitarium.

There are a great many doctors and nutritionists today who recommend a vegetarian diet for all heart sufferers.

STROKES

Every year hundreds of thousands of people become victims of strokes. Although this disorder is frequently associated with the later years of life, this is not necessarily an affliction of old age. A few years ago, for example, a wellknown English motion picture actress in her late thirties had a stroke.

A stroke occurs when the blood supply to a part of the brain is reduced or completely cut off. When the nerve cells in that part of the brain are deprived of oxygen and blood supply, they cannot function ... and the part of the body controlled by these nerve cells cannot function, either. The results of a stroke depend upon the part of the brain which is affected and the seriousness or extent of the damage. A stroke can be fatal. It can produce paralysis of one entire side of the body or a portion of the body or a single part. A "lighter" stroke may cause difficulty in moving the arms or legs or in speaking, or may result in loss of memory.

After a stroke, the damaged nerve cells may recover, or their functions may be taken over by other brain cells. Some victims may suffer such serious damage that it will take a long time to make even a partial recovery.

108

Immediate attention to proper diet and exercise can do much toward helping the stroke victim regain the use of affected muscles. Physical therapy treatment should be begun as soon as possible to aid rehabilitation and help speed recovery. Prolonged inactivity impairs the circulation and makes recovery more difficult.

A stroke usually originates from the same causes as a heart attack. The arteries become clogged and narrow by deposits of cholesterol and minerals in the arterial walls, hindering the free passage of the blood. Pressure of the bloodstream trying to force its way through further irritates the walls of the arteries, helping to create conditions for formation of blood clots. When a clot breaks off from the lining of the artery wall into the bloodstream, it can block the flow of blood completely.

If complete blockage occurs in vital arteries that feed the heart muscle, the result is a heart attack or coronary thrombosis. If this disaster occurs in the cerebral arteries of the brain, it causes a stroke, sometimes called "a heart attack in the head."

BRIGHT'S DISEASE

When the small arteries of the kidneys are affected, the condition produced is known as "dropsy" or Bright's disease. The most noticeable symptoms are swelling of the ankles and legs. Although swollen ankles and legs (known as edema of these parts) does not always indicate Bright's disease, this ailment is so widespread and insidious that it must be suspected and a physician consulted.

Whether the thickening and blocking process takes place in the heart, head or kidneys, it is essentially the same disease. Doctors refer to it as atheroslerosis. This means that the arteries that carry the blood are blocked with the hard, waxy substance known as cholesterol.

Let me impress upon you that *prevention is far better than cure*, and generally more successful. That is why I keep stressing proper diet and exercise. Get it completely out of your head that years alone bring damage to the heart and

109

blood vessels. Remember that age is not toxic, and that age is not a force but a measure. Live so that you will never get a stroke. Live so that you will never get a heart attack. You know what your enemies are—tobacco, overweight (unhealthy fat), stimulants such as coffee and tea, alcohol and cola drinks, fatty foods, salt and salty foods, lack of daily exercise.

FOLLOW THIS HEART FITNESS PROGRAM

This Heart Fitness Program is designed to help you have a stronger heart and build a "youthful" circulation. Nature cannot be pushed or rushed . . . but if you will cooperate with her vital power, you can have "the heart of a lion."

If you have a weak heart, weak "pipes" that are clogged and corroded, remember that it took you a long time to get them in that condition . . . and you must be patient with Nature while the regeneration and rejuvenation processes take place within your body.

A fit "youthful" heart can be yours if you are willing to work for it. No one else can make your heart strong. It depends upon YOU. Your eating habits and your physical activity will determine the type of heart you have.

POSITIVE THINKING AND POSITIVE ACTION

To have a strong and powerful heart you must develop strong willpower. You must overcome all negative thoughts about the human heart. Do not let cowards and weaklings influence you away from following your Heart Fitness Program. These fear mongers will try to impart their fear to you, telling you that exercise will strain your heart and that after reaching a certain age you should confine your activities to a rocking chair. Don't believe them!

In following this Heart Fitness Program you are working with Science and Nature. Don't let unqualified people influence you away from it. Many years of research and investigation have gone into the development of this Heart Fitness Program, in order to give you a master plan for building a strong, fit heart and a long, healthy life.

110

MY SIX POINTS

I have written this book not so much to help you as to help you help yourself. If I repeat certain points, it is with the zeal with which one taps a nail already driven home. My main objective in these pages is to inspire you with a more intense enthusiasm for health, and to warn you against certain dangers which you may easily overlook.

In a Brotherly Way I Have Tried To Stress These Points:

1. You have but one heart and one life and you should take care of these treasures.

2. Your body must obey the commands of your mind. Flesh is dumb.

3. Every bad habit that weakens your heart and shortens your life must be banished.

4. You should demand of yourself a higher standard of health and happiness.

5. You should regard your body as a fine instrument or precision machine whose care and control is in your hands.

6. With increasing years you should draw closer and closer to Nature and simplify your life.

Let us, then, throw ourselves on Nature, try to understand her, follow her laws, and live as it would seem she wants us to live. She may be cruel and kill us at times ... but civilization kills us twice as fast.

Lukewarm water will not take a locomotive anywhere, nor will lukewarm purpose lift a man to any noticeable height of achievement.

THE COMPLETE NATURIST

The ideal of the Complete Naturist is to identify himself so completely with Nature that he becomes part and parcel of her. He lives simply. He lets the earth, air and sun work their will with him. With serene, clear-eyed confidence he puts himself into Nature's hands, lets her run his machine, heal his hurts, comfort him in sickness and adversity ... then when his usefulness to her is ended, lets her call him back home.

Let your body be nourished by natural food and rain water or distilled water, fresh air and sunlight. Exercise it and relax it, and leave Nature to do the rest. Treat your body with the same care and wisdom that you would a valued animal of purebred stock ... and as surely as your animal will take prizes, so will you. It is easy to sneer at "health-minded, back-to-nature" people ... but we who believe in Nature will have the last laugh.

GET CLOSE TO THE EARTH

It is good to establish contact with the earth, to let your bare feet grip the living rock, to feel the soft mud and squish it between your toes. I love to take sun and air baths, to lie on my back gripping the green grass and staring into the blue abyss of the sky. I love to lie on the beach beside a sea or lake or river, with as little clothing on as permissable. Clothing is a non-conductor of earth electricity. Only through the naked skin can that most subtle of currents pass. Discard all the clothing possible and let sun, air and water have their way with you. Keep in close touch with Mother Earth, letting her strength and virtue pass into you through the bare soles of your feet.

Civilization has complicated our lives with hot-house living. Man was a healthier, happier creature when he lived close to Nature. Just stand on any street of any big city and watch the people frantically rushing past. From your standard of High Health you will see that three out of four of them are probably sick or physically unfit. Very rarely do you see one of superlative health.

112

GET THE FEELING OF NATURE

Don't be like the average sick or half-sick person. They have never known the real thrill of living. Most humans today are addicted to some kind of dope such as tobacco, coffee, tea, alcohol, cola drinks ... and in many instances they are "hooked" on some kind of narcotic, mild or strong. People turn to dope when their vitality hits the bottom level. When health is gone, vitality goes with it and so does the zest for living. In a desperate effort to get "kicks" out of life these poor creatures turn to dope.

In the old days it used to be the middle-aged and the oldsters who felt they had to seek dope or other artificial means to hang onto life. Now, tragically, young people are using dope and drugs of all kinds. They are throwing away their natural vitality, turning their backs on Nature. They are candidates for heart attacks. The heart is damaged by all forms of stimulants and depressants.

The further we get away from living according to the Laws of Nature, the sicker we get both physically and mentally.

One of the dominant suggestions of this book for building a powerful heart at any age is a gradual return to a more natural form of living. In food, exercise, breathing, sleeping, clothing and simplicity of life ... try to reach a closeness to Nature that makes you almost one with her. You will never have a weak, sick heart when you live close to Mother Nature and in partnership with her. When you can feel that the same pure and elemental forces that express themselves in a pine tree are also expressing themselves in you, you have made big strides toward a health ideal.

Begin to live as Nature wants you to live. Seek to feel that she claims you, and that you are a part of all glad, growing things. Put yourself into Nature's hands as they do.

Know that Nature is eager to aid you. She can run that ill-used machine of yours better than any other agency, human or divine. And when it breaks down in her hands, it is because its usefulness is at an end.

Dear friend, I wish above all things that thou may prosper and be in health even as the soul prosper—3 John:2

THE ART OF LIVING LONG

One of the best recipes for a long life is just to keep on living. There is no substitute for LIFE!

Consider each day a little life in itself, and make it as perfect and well rounded as you can. Try to have a stronger heart and better health on your next birthday than you have today. In living supremely for the moment you are living superbly for the future.

But you must always be aware of yourself. The moment you relax your guard the enemy is ready to rush in and smite you in your heart. True, you may live long without trying to ... but you will live longer if you make the effort. Living for longevity is an art. The man who deliberately sets himself to prolong his days has a healthy chance of doing so.

Forgetfulness of self may make the time go like magic, but it does not help build a strong heart and keep you youthful. It means inattention to yourself and consequent carelessness. As you live longer you should grow less objective and more subjective. The more self-centered you are, the better you will conserve yourself. Generally speaking, it is not the self-sacrificing but the selfish who are granted the long life ... not those who forget themselves in others, but those who are most conscious of themselves.

This may seem to give a ruthless character to longevity. Not at all! Eating is ruthless, but without nourishment we cannot aspire to fulfill our dreams. To seek selfishly to prolong one's life is to extend one's term of human usefulness. I am not advocating that you prolong your own life at the expense of others ... but that you live a long and healthy life so that you may be useful to others as well as to yourself.

The secret of longevity is to understand that *the enemy is not age but aging,* and to put up a strong defense against it. Some people, of course, are born with such wonderful constitutions that they simply can't kill themselves. You will find octogenarians who tell you that they owe their long life to smoking, alcohol and no exercise. You can tell them just as confidently that they could extend their life span by a good twenty years by taking better care of their health.

114

LONGEVITY IS RESISTANCE

Scientific longevity is organized resistance. It is based on a knowledge of the body and of the laws of health. Above all, it means reliance on Nature. Nature abhors ill health, which is another name for poisoning. She is always striving to purify, to vitalize. She wants to help you if you will only let her. Drugs and doctors will do you no good if Nature is not backing them up.

HEART AND BLOOD VESSEL DISEASES
ARE YOUR GREATEST THREAT

In the fight before you, remember that you must defend yourself against coronary thrombosis (heart attack), stroke, hypertension (high blood pressure), arteriosclerosis (hardening of the arteries), atherosclerosis (blockage and clogging of the arteries by cholesterol and other debris), angina pectoris, varicose veins, and other cardio-vascular (heart and blood vessel) diseases.

Diseases of the heart and blood vessels, as we have noted, are the *No. 1 Killer in the United States* taking more than a million American lives each year—more than all other causes combined.

You must also wage war against stiffening joints, fibrous tissues, deafness, blindness and many other enemies of health and life.

All this means that there must be little relaxing of your activity. The advice to "grow old gracefully" is, I believe, quite wrong. Time will force you to do so in the end when Nature says so ... but until then, it is far better to grow old strenuously. Put up a valiant resistance! *You are "as old as you feel"* ... so *FEEL YOUNG*! If you abide by Nature's Laws, you can't help feeling young. By trusting in Nature, obeying her laws, understanding your physical machine and how to care for it, you can live a long, long life.

It seems to me that what we call "old age" is the result of sluggish cell action in the body. The cells are being renewed all the time by the moisture in the lymph circulation, just as a tree is renewed all the time by the circulation of its sap. But if the cell is clogged in any way by deposits which it cannot completely get rid of—chiefly because of poor circulation of the blood—it cannot use to full advantage the material brought for its renewal by the lymph or the nourishment and oxygen delivered by the blood.

In reporting an address given recently by *Dr. W. M. Malisoff, professor of biochemistry at Brooklyn Polytechnic Institute*, the Associated Press quotes: "On the basis of what we have done with rabbits, we have come to the conclusion that if we can do the same thing for man, he can live a healthy and normal life until the age 185 ... A waxy material, cholesterol, is deposited on the arteries and there is a correlation between age and the amount of cholesterol deposited ... In tests of 52 rabbits, we have been able to reverse the symptoms of old age."

Biologists tell us that man grows an entirely new body every 11 months. That being the case, why does it take on the appearance of age? Scientists answer this by saying that it fails to shed all of the old. As I stated before, deposits in the cell prevent its full use of the renewal material. So, instead of living 7 times the period it takes him to mature as animals do, man's life is proportionately much shorter.

Confirmation of this statement comes from *Dr. Serge Veronoff of Paris, France*, who says that each of us should live to be 140 years old. A human being is matured at 20 years of age. Nature constructed the human machine to live 7 times that age, or 140 years. The fact that some men and women even today have been able to reach and surpass the age of 120 years and have then died of disease seems to prove the validity of a normal 140-year life span.

Deposits in the arteries retard the circulation of the blood. The speed and efficiency of the blood has much to do with the prolongation of life. It is the current of blood which provides the entire body with the required nourishment and oxygen, and removes harmful substances for elimination. Slowing of blood circulation, loss of elasticity of the blood vessels and any disturbances of the machinery which regulates distribution of blood are among the most important causes of shortening of life, vigor and health.

116

In my opinion, there is no physiological principle limiting life or health. I believe that youthfulness and radiant health can be self-controlled.

This is your life. It is your duty to yourself to learn how to keep the body healthy for a long life.

THE MAIN CAUSE OF WIDOWHOOD IS CORONARY DISEASE IN MEN

The number one cause of widowhood in the United States is coronary (heart) disease in men. Remember our discussion of cholesterol earlier in this book . . . and that high cholesterol levels are an invitation to heart attack. Statistics show that cholesterol levels in American men increase rapidly between ages 30 and 65. Be on guard! Have your blood cholesterol level test twice a year.

Women before the age of 50 prove to be much better protected against degenerative artery disease than men. After 50, however, women begin to develop heart attacks and strokes with the same frequency as men. The scientific conclusion is that female sex hormones play an important part in providing protection against the menace of atherosclerosis. As soon as the change of life starts in women, the protection of these sex hormones apparently ceases, and they become equally as susceptible as men to heart attacks and strokes. This does not mean, however, that women under 50 should neglect the care of their hearts, because there are plenty of exceptions to the rule . . . thousands of women do have heart attacks and strokes before the age of 50.

MODERN MAN DOES NOT DIE . . . HE COMMITS SLOW SUICIDE

Just because you are *"feeling fine"* does not mean that you can afford the risk of continuing to choke your bloodstream with the high cholesterol diet typical of most people in our western civilization. Ham and eggs, meat and potatoes, pies and cakes, bread with butter or margarine, milk and ice cream . . . all the rich foods that most men and many women dote on

117

... are slow poisons to your heart and circulatory system. Remember that these poisons work silently and insidiously. Their effect may not become evident until you suddenly have a heart attack.

But remember the wise words of Dr. Dudley White—that death from a heart attack is not sudden ... it's been building up for years.

WIVES—YOUR HUSBAND'S LIFE IS IN YOUR HANDS

I would like to suggest to all wives that you re-read Dr. White's warning (page 26) ... and that you take it seriously. If you want to keep your husbands alive ... work on them to exercise every day, and watch what you feed them and yourself. You may be shortening the lives of your husband and your family with too many fattening and highly saturated foods. Their lives are in YOUR HANDS. You prepare and put the food on the table for the family to eat. You will learn from this valuable book how to keep your family in perfect health ... and you and your family will soon discover a startling increase in vigor and vitality, with a sense of wellbeing.

Remember young people also can die of heart trouble. So teach your children how to eat correctly. Give your family more fresh salads, more lightly steamed vegetables, more fresh fruit desserts. Ration the butter at each meal. Serve your meat lean and rare ... and leave off the gravy (it's loaded with cholesterol). Limit the amount of dairy products. Remember, adults do not need milk! Serve them delicious herb teas such as mint, alfalfa, anise seed. Banish coffee from your table. And throw away the salt shaker!

Your reward will be a happy, healthy family.

There are three Bragg Health Books which you will find very helpful in planning your overall health-building diet. These are: "Healthful Eating Without Confusion," "Bragg's Complete Health Gourmet Recipes For Vital Health," and our "Vegetarian Gourmet Health Recipes (no salt, no sugar). (Please see back pages for ordering.)

Everything in excess is opposed by nature. —Hippocrates

EAT YOUR BIGGEST MEAL IN THE MIDDLE OF THE DAY

It seems to be an American custom for people to eat the biggest meal in the evening. From a standpoint of heart attacks, this is the worst time to eat a big meal, especially a meal with a preponderance of fat. It has been definitely established by research scientists that the blood is more likely to clot 2 to 8 hours following a meal with a high fat intake. It would therefore seem desirable to avoid heavy meals, particularly in the evening, to minimize the chances of intravascular clotting. The occurence of coronary thrombosis after the eating of a heavy meal has been familiar to doctors for years. How often we read or hear about a man in his prime dying of a heart attack during his sleep at night!

Retired people, of course, can regulate their mealtimes easily. Business people can dine at an earlier hour in the evening, and can certainly regulate their diet to promote their health and prolong their lives.

The ideal meal for evening is completely vegetarian. It can begin with a raw combination salad with lemon and oil dressing, followed by two cooked vegetables such as stringbeans, Italian squash (zucchini), peas, corn on the cob, kale, okra, vegetable chop suey, etc. Several nights a week add a baked potato—but do not drench this potato in fat! Season with sea kelp or any tasty herb and safflower, soy or olive oil instead of butter.

Now I am not telling you that the price we must pay to avoid a heart attack and live a longer life is to give up the pleasures of good food. Far from it! As I told you earlier, *delicious French dishes* that are world famous are *among the best anti-coronary recipes*. A good French chef rarely uses salt and pepper and cooks with very little fat. The secrets of French flavor lie in the skillful use of herbs, garlic, onions, green peppers, mushrooms and the like.

Now learn what and how great benefits a temperate diet will bring along with it. In the first place, you will enjoy good health. —Horace 65 B.C.

DELICIOUS CHINESE RECIPES PROMOTE HEART HEALTH

Americans have ten times as high a coronary rate as the Chinese. The Chinese have a low cholesterol, low fat diet—in sharp contrast to the high cholesterol, high fat diet found in the United States, Canada and the more prosperous countries of Europe. Pathologists, scientists and medical researchers have produced overwhelming evidence that when blood cholesterol and fats are high, the arteries are also in the same degree of atherosclerosis. *Atherosclerosis has always been a "disease of the affluent"*—only those who could afford rich, fatty foods have been victims of heart attack and stroke. Cholesterol was found in the arteries of the mummies of the Pharoahs of Egypt, whose diet was far richer than that of their subjects. The degenerative diseases of the heart and blood vessels have traditionally and historically been associated with royalty and the "wealthy classes."

Today, however, we have millions and millions of people in our western industrialized countries who can afford the rich foods of royalty. You hear and read about "the affluent society" and its blessings. But this affluence is exacting a high price in atherosclerosis and the fast rising epidemic of heart attacks and strokes.

Hundreds of millions of peoples living in China and other Asian countries in a non-affluent society are rarely afflicted with heart disease. One of the main items of their diet is—and has been for centuries—one of the most healthful of all vegetable oils, soy oil. Soy oil contains a high percentage of unsaturated fatty acids and lecithin, two of the most protective factors against heart disease.

The basic Chinese diet is rice and lightly cooked vegetables, with meat used only as an occasional flavoring. When you order chicken or beef chop suey in a Chinese restaurant, you get a plentiful dish of vegetables such as celery, onions, green bellpeppers, bamboo shoots, water chestnuts and bean sprouts, and only a very small amount of finely sliced chicken or beef. With this you get a dish of rice. No bread and butter is served at an authentic Chinese restaurant.

Thy food shall be thy remedy.—Hippocrates

120

At my home we are very fond of Chinese food. Here are the recipes of our favorite Chinese meal, which we have several times a week:

Raw Combination Salad

Break lettuce into bite-size pieces. Add sliced celery (greener the better), radishes, carrots and cucumbers, tomatoes, and fresh chopped parsley and spinach. Toss with a dressing of soy or safflower oil and fresh lemon or orange juice.

Mushroom Chop Suey

With a sharp knife slice onions, green bellpeppers, celery, chard, carrots, cabbage and any other vegetables you are to add. Mix with bean sprouts (fresh or canned), water chestnuts, bamboo shots (fresh or canned) and mushrooms (fresh or canned).

Put these mixed vegetables into a wok or skillet and add a small amount of unsaturated oil such as olive, corn, soy or safflower oil. Fresh sliced garlic may be added if you enjoy it. (We do. We feel that garlic helps purify the body's pipes and helps boost your immune system.) Just before serving stir in 1-2 teaspoons of Bragg Liquid Aminos, or you may spray it over the vegetable mix just before serving for a delicious Oriental soy sauce flavor.

The secret of Chinese food is not to overcook it. Saute this chop suey mixture 5 to 10 minutes at the very most, stirring constantly with a wooden spoon.

If you eat meat, you may add a small amount of chicken, lean beef or shrimp to the chop suey vegetables—but remember, just a small amount and sliced very thin.

Brown Rice

Brown rice is a healthy staple. Use natural brown rice — 1 cup to 3 cups distilled water. Add 1/2 teaspoon Bragg Liquid Aminos and 1 teaspoon olive oil. Cook in a double boiler or in a thick-bottomed pan with a tight lid over medium heat until rice is soft and fluffy. Do not stir until ready to serve. Just before serving you may add a dash or spray of Bragg Liquid Aminos for even a more delicious flavor. This makes 3-4 generous servings.

Dessert

A fresh apple, pear, banana or other fresh fruit tops off this perfect anti-coronary meal. _____

The chemistry of the food a person eats becomes his own body chemistry.

YOU CAN TEACH OLD DOGS NEW TRICKS

They say you cannot teach an old dog new tricks. But I believe that mature humans have the intelligence to protect themselves against heart attacks by learning new tricks of eating. Isn't it worth it to know that you are not going to wake up in the middle of the night gasping for air and clutching your heart?

To avoid heart attacks you must learn to substitute the natural vegetable oils (*unsaturated fats) for butter, margarine and other saturated and hydrogenated fats. If you are a milk drinker, you must then learn to make "milk" with soya powder and drink that instead of cow's milk. You must learn to use herbs, kelp, garlic, onions and other natural ingredients to impart delicious and distinctive flavor and aroma instead of salting your food. * *Keep to bare minimum needs.*

Most people shake their heads in doubt when told they must give up the use of salt in cooking. It does take a little time to make the change-over from salt to natural, nourishing herbs and kelp. But, as I have told you, the craving for salt is acquired and not natural, and it will disappear, just as mine did. You will find that your 260 taste buds, like mine, will reject salted foods.

You know now that the saturated fats in meats, eggs and dairy products are your enemies. You must learn to use them most sparingly.

It's your life ... the only one you have. It's your heart ... you only get one good one. Remember, when you satisfy an overly demanding appetite for health-destroying foods, you are actually helping to destroy your best and essential vital organ—your own heart!

Perhaps the most valuable result of all education is the ability to make yourself do the thing you have to do, when it ought to be done, as it ought to be done, whether you like to do it or not.

STOP HEART TROUBLE BEFORE IT STARTS

I believe it is far better to make a few changes in the diet than to drag around a paralyzed arm or leg or both as the result of a stroke ... or to have your life cut short by a heart attack.

So, stop this very minute for a meditation period and have a heart to heart talk with yourself. Make up your mind that you are not going to die with a heart attack or be crippled by a stroke. Life is the survival of the fittest ... and no one—yes, no one!—is going to be able to protect your heart except yourself! It's your duty to yourself to live so that your heart can remain strong and powerful throughout your entire natural life span.

We must live by knowledge and wisdom and not by old wives' tales and myths. This is why this book was written ... to give you the scientific facts about your heart and a Heart Fitness Program that will tell you how to take care of it.

This book is simple. It truthfully tells what a heart attack is, what causes it, and what you can start doing today to prevent it. I have no magic formula or cure for heart trouble. In this Heart Fitness Program I have simply brought together well documented evidence from the great scientific and medical researchers and statisticians of the world.

Today the world is turning toward heart transplants. I am not the least interested in heart transplants. Nor am I interested in the diagnosis and treatment of heart troubles. I am interested in PREVENTION by keeping the heart fit and healthy. Let's stop heart troubles before they start! Why wait for the heart to deteriorate before we do something about it?

Today we must live so that we do not have a heart attack in the future. What we sow in one period of our lives, we reap in another. Let's sow the seeds of good health and we will automatically have a powerful and fit heart.

Your birthday is the beginning of your own personal new year. Your first birthday was a beginning, and each new birthday is a chance to begin again, to start over, to take a new grip on life. — **Paul C. Bragg**

FEEL YOUNG REGARDLESS OF YOUR BIRTHDAYS

We can definitely capture the joyous feeling of youthfu[l]ness no matter what our calendar years may be. By living t[he] Health-Life as outlined in this Heart Fitness Program, we ca[n] again feel the joy of feeling youthful.

Don't let "Old" people drag you down to their level [of] thinking, "*You are as young as your arteries.*" And you a[re] going to live a healthful life so you can help keep the arteri[es] youthful. Keep your arteries young and your thinking your[g] and you will feel young!

Age is not a matter of birthdays, it is a matter of how we[ll] you feel.

ONE OF MY YOUTHFUL FRIENDS IS ROY D. WHITE, 10[6]

Roy just celebrated his 106th birthday—yes, you rea[d] correctly—106 years young! Roy D. White lives in Lor[g] Beach, California. He has a keen brain, a great sense [of] humor and a feeling of youthfulness tingling throughout h[is] supple, straight and active body. Roy can put both han[ds] over head, keep his knees stiff and bend over and touch h[is] toes—an exercise people half his age cannot do. And he nev[er] fails to walk his five miles a day. Being a widower, Roy tak[es] care of his own apartment and prepares all his own meals. A[t] 106, he appears to be a youthful active 75 with the physic[al] agility of a man many years younger.

Remember throughout this Heart Fitness Program I hav[e] told you how important it is to keep physically alive. And it [is] backed up by this 106 year old youngster. You cannot let th[e] circulation slow down ... *to rest is to rust and rust* [is] *destruction.*

Roy believes long walks help you physically, mentally an[d] spiritually. Roy believes you can walk off your tensions an[d] worries. Roy says, "*I've always been free from tensions—that's the foundation of my Philosophy of Life. Fear an[d] hatred are the two worst things in the world. You can multi[p]ly your troubles by thinking they are worse than they ar[e] and no matter how mean anyone has been to me, I've nev[er] hated them. Let them do the hating.*"

124

Tensions, anger and excessive emotionalism all can help damage your heart.

Roy has the great philosophy of forgiving and forgetting. He says that children and young people think that way and he wants to always think young.

You and I know that when you have such a sense of well-being and feel youthful, your entire attitude toward life is fresher and more youthful. One's whole philosophy can change to a younger, more optimistic one, in place of the stagnating and defeatist attitude that so many older people have. When you feel youthful, you act youthful; and above all you think youthful.

IT'S NEVER TOO LATE TO THINK YOUTHFUL

This whole Heart Fitness Program is to make you forget birthdays and live a youthful, carefree life. This feeling and philosophy of life prevents many physical and mental miseries that are especially apt to afflict older people. In this way you can maintain health, strength, vigor and happiness as the years roll by. It has been said that "There is really no cure for old age; only those who die young escape it." But this Heart Fitness Program can really help you feel younger, as you live longer.

I NO LONGER CELEBRATE BIRTHDAYS

That is absolutely right. No more birthdays for me! I no longer want to measure my life by calendar years—only biological years.

Yes, I have more than my three score and ten. Yes, I am a great great grandfather. But I am not going to stop from enjoying my youthful activities. I am going to continue to play tennis with the youngsters, climb the mountains with the mountain climbers, swim with the swimmers and dance with the pretty young girls—the senior girls who are still young in heart. One of my favorite dancing partners is a girl only 88— but oh, what a dancer! She is as graceful as any of my great-granddaughters.

Don't think the years are making you old—it's the way you live that damages your heart and clogs your arteries.

You must earn your bonus years, you must earn your youthful arteries ... you must work hard to preserve the vitality and the fitness of your heart. And the wonderful part of it is that when you build up a fit heart and body, you find the time for so many more activities than you did when you were dragging around half-alive. When you have a heart that is ticking joyfully, the world looks like the Garden of Eden. You become a carefree person with a song in your heart, a sparkle in your eye and a spring in your step. Life can be beautiful—for when you are healthy, you are happy. And after all is that not the greatest goal in life—sweet, contented HAPPINESS!

NOW GET TO WORK

Start this very minute on your Heart Fitness Program! Get it firmly in your mind that you are going to build a fit heart. Banish all negative thoughts. Have faith ... for you are now going to work with a powerful force, Mother Nature. Say to yourself day after day, "I am building a good, strong, fit heart." Think strength and vitality of the heart.

You must be master of yourself at all times. You are surely more powerful than that cup of coffee, more forceful than tobacco, alcohol, salt, fat and other toxic substances that help to destroy the heart. Take command of your body and mind today ... this minute ... and let nothing distract you from adhering to your Heart Fitness Program.

If you feel yourself weakening in your resolve, look to a Higher Power for courage and willpower. You were given one heart ... one body ... one life by your Creator, and you were given Nature as your ally to help you achieve a long, healthy and happy life. But no one, not even Nature, can help you unless you help yourself. Now get to work!

Wisdom is the principal thing; therefore get wisdom: and with all thy getting get understanding. — Proverbs 4:7

CHELATION THERAPY

THE "MIRACLE" METHOD OF UNCLOGGING THE ARTERIES

We want to share with you a miracle of medical science which we recently learned about and found so amazing that we checked into it thoroughly. We have found impressive clinical medical evidence, borne out by our own personal investigation, that a safe, reliable therapeutic method has been developed to counteract the ravages of the degenerative diseases -- so prevalent in our society today -- that arise from hardening and clogging of the arteries (arteriosclerosis and atherosclerosis) . . . which cause heart attacks and strokes. The heart attack is the No. 1 killer in the United States today!

This method is known as Chelation (pronouced key-lation) Therapy. It has proved effective to the point of being termed "miraculous" by physicians as well as patients.

"Miraculous isn't the word -- it's incredible!" declared J., the first chelation therapy patient we interviewed.

We met J. through a mutual friend, Attorney Kirkpatrick W. Dilling of Chicago, who was visiting us in Desert Hot Springs, California, and insisted that we go to J.'s home in nearby Palm Desert to learn firsthand of his recent "miracle".

Only six months ago a leading heart specialist had told J., a man in his forties, that he had a life expectancy of two years unless he underwent drastic surgery for a "3-way bypass" -- i.e., transplanting blood vessels from his leg into his heart to bridge or "bypass" blockage in three arteries (with 100%, 95% and 75% blockage). If he survived the surgery, there was no guarantee that similar blockage would not recur. J. was in despair.

Through the National Health Federation, he learned about Ray Evers, M.D., who for a number of years has been achieving remarkable recoveries in such cases with chelation therapy. Average treatment period is three to four weeks and you can be an out-patient in any of the doctor's offices or clinics that administer chelation therapy. So J. began an eight-week series of treatments.

When we met him, three months after he had entered Dr. Evers' hospital, J. had just undergone a stress and thermogram test at Loma Linda ... and there was no indication of any heart or circulatory problems whatever. J. was jubilant!

A must-read book about life-saving chelation therapy ... it's an eye-opener on how to never need a bypass and why you would not want one! It's called "Bypassing Bypass" by Elmer M. Cranton, M.D., and you can order it through Health Science for $9.95 plus $1.50 shipping. See back pages for book order form.

REVERSAL OF THE "AGING PROCESS"

Shortly thereafter, we went to visit Dr. Evers (now retired) at Meadowbrook Hospital in Belle Chasse, Lousiana. He told us that over seven years he treated more than 7,000 patients with chelation therapy. He said that he believed chelation therapy "could hold the key to the basic treatment of some of mankind's greatest killer diseases, all characterized by the same basic abnormality — that is, narrowing and closing off of the blood vessels, which can affect every organ of the body."

"Everyone is familiar with the clinical picture of coronary or heart attacks and strokes or brain clots and hemorrhages," he continued, "but many other diseases such as diabetes, thyroid and adrenal disturbances, digestive problems, senility, emphysema, arthritis, multiple sclerosis, etc., may also be caused, at least in part, by interference with the proper delivery of blood to vital structures.

"Chelation therapy attacks this basic problem of the cardiovascular system," Dr. Evers pointed out. "The results often produce significant relief of symptoms, are often life saving and sometimes miraculous."

"We saw proof of his words with our own eyes. We saw people from their 40's to their 80's being brought into the hospital in wheelchairs . . . the victims of heart attacks and other heart and circulatory ailments, strokes, diabetic gangrene, crippling arthritis, senility, and similar degenerative diseases . . . and several weeks later we saw these same people walking out of the hospital with a spring in their step, aglow with the joy of living.

What brought about this amazing rejuvenation?

The arteries of these people were being unclogged by chelation therapy . . . cleansed of the accumulated debris that had hardened and thickened the walls of these vital blood vessels. Now the "pipes" were being opened, and once more the blood (the river of life) could course through arteries, veins and capillaries to bring life-giving oxygen and nourishment to every cell in the body and carry off toxic wastes.

The process of degeneration . . . commonly called the "aging process" . . . was being reversed.

Sad Facts: 25% of hospital deaths are due to medical doctors errors. Play safe — before any chemical, drug treatments (chemo, etc...) or serious surgery, it is best to get 2 to 3 evaluations to be positive you are making a right decision for your future health! Once treatment or surgery is done — is often too late to make amends — so the time to get consultation is before, not after the fact! It is your body and your right to help and judge in all decisions of your health and future well being!

WHAT CAUSES "AGING?"

As we have already discussed in this book, the so-called "aging process" is not the result of the passage of time . . . it is primarily the result of inadequate blood circulation, which can and does occur at any calendar age.

The chief villains are *an excess of inorganic calcium, of which undistilled drinking water is a primary source,* and an excess of cholesterol from a diet rich in saturated animal fats and hydrogenated fats.

Arteriosclerosis, or hardening of the arteries, results from calcium deposits in the arterial walls. In atherosclerosis, the calcified walls are further thickened by deposits of cholesterol, dangerously narrowing the passageway of the blood.

The calcium seems to act as a cementing agent, forming plaques with the cholesterol, to which other inorganic minerals and waxlike fats attach themselves. The narrowing of the lumen or passageway lessens both the quantity and the force of the blood flow. Body cells degenerate from lack of nourishment and their own toxicity, and a number of them die.

WHAT IS CHELATION THERAPY?

Chelation therapy is a therapeutic adaptation of a natural biochemical process.

The term "chelation" derives from the Greek word *chele* (pronounced keely) meaning a crab-like claw. Without going into the detailed chemistry, chelation in human metabolism is the process by which an enzyme grabs or "binds" an organic mineral or "metal" and transports it to the part of the body where it can be utilized . . . zinc to the pancreas for the manufacture of insulin, for example; iron for the hemoglobin (red blood cells); calcium for building bones and for its many other uses in the body; etc. (Remember, this refers to organic calcium -- not inorganic, which cannot be used.)

This natural chelation process was not discovered and explained in biochemical research until the early 1940's. Its first therapeutic application was during World War II with the creation of a synthetic chelating agent that would act as an antidote for "mustard gas" (lewisite) and other forms of arsenic poisoning. For some 20 years thereafter, chelating agents were developed almost exclusively for ridding the body of toxic heavy metals such as lead. The chelation process was also used in industry, in the manufacture of detergents and petroleum products.

During the late 1950's it was discovered that chelating agents used as poison antidotes were also effective in removing inorganic calcium deposits from joints, organs and the cardiovascular system of the human body, and special studies were begun in this field.

Through careful biochemical and clinical medical research, a safe and very effective chelating agent, known as EDTA, was produced for the specific purpose of chelating inorganic calcium from living tissues and transporting it for excretion through the kidneys and bowels. The EDTA formula perfected for medical use is Endrate disodium (Abbott).

EDTA or Endrate does not affect the normal organic calcium utilized by the body, but chelates only pathological calcium deposits. It unclogs the arteries by chelating the calcium out of the atherosclerotic plaques, which then break up. The cholesterol and other deposits become slushy and are flushed out through the bloodstream. All the residue "goes down the drain" and the "pipes" become open and free flowing.

THERAPY INCLUDES PROPER DIET AND SUPPLEMENTS

Carlos P. Lamar, M.D., F.I.C.A., of Coral Gables, Florida, a pioneer in chelation therapy since 1960, developed the basic procedures which have been followed so successfully to date. These include the proper dosage of Endrate, the slow intravenous method of administration, which varies from 2½ to 4 hours per treatment, as well as the initial periods of treatment and follow-up therapy for various conditions.

As an essential part of chelation treatment, Dr. Lamar and his colleagues prescribe an anti-atherogenic diet, avoiding large meals in favor of more frequent, lighter meals, with total elimination of dairy foods (which contain both calcium and cholesterol) and a sharp restriction of saturated fat. Emphasis is placed on live foods. (And we would like to add that drinking and cooking water should be only steam distilled water.)

A minimum vitamin supplement of 100 mg of Vitamin B6 (pyridoxine) is included in the diet, with additional vitamin and/or mineral supplements as required by the individual patient. During treatment, the patient is allowed as much freedom of mobility as possible.

SAFE DIAGNOSIS BY THERMOGRAM

All patients are given thorough physical and laboratory examinations before the start of chelation therapy, carefully

130

monitored during the course of treatment, and given complete instruction for follow-up procedures.

We were particularly impressed with a marvelous new invention in diagnostic equipment . . . the thermograph . . . which provides a completely safe and accurate method of locating and determining the degree of arterial blockage. Formerly this had to be done by the angiogram test, often at great risk to the patient.

The thermograph is a heat sensitive instrument which records bodily heat in direct correlation to blood circulation. The thermogram of the patient reveals any and all blockage, its precise location . . . and the degree of the blockage, indicated by a light spectrum with a ten-color range.

We have never recommended taking the risk of an angiogram . . . but we do endorse the thermogram without reservation.

CHELATION THERAPY PROMOTES NATURAL HEALING

Because it attacks the basic cardiovascular problem of degeneration, chelation therapy helps regenerate the body's natural self-healing and self-repairing powers. The restoration of normal blood circulation restores normal metabolism and biochemical functions. The whole body "comes alive".

This is why chelation therapy, from the very beginning, has exceeded medical expectations.

When the first cases were reported in 1964 by Dr. Lamar, in the national medical publication *Angiology* (Vol. 15, No. 9, Sept. 1964), the most surprising result was the significant decrease in the insulin requirement of diabetics in response to chelation therapy. Two of the early cases were "hopeless" elderly diabetics with severe cardiovascular complications and mental deterioration. There was a complete remission of symptoms, both physical and mental, plus the marked decrease in the insulin requirement. This "bonus" was attributed to the increased circulation in the pancreas, promoting normal insulin production.

Since then, chelation therapy has been found to achieve such "bonus benefits" as regeneration and rehardening of softened bone areas in osteoporosis, restoration of mobility to frozen osteoarthritic joints, clearing up of prostatic calcinosis, relief from hypothyroidism, recovery of normal kidney function, as well as normal function in other glands and organs, visual improvement in deteriorated retinas -- in fact, improvement in all pathological conditions resulting from impaired circulation.

131

Chelation treatment with Endrate has proved effective as an antidote to snake venom. It has achieved marked improvement in patients suffering from those two baffling diseases of the central nervous system, multiple sclerosis and Parkinson's disease.

Perhaps the most spectacular results of chelation therapy are evident in the restoration of mental acuity in cases of advanced senility. As Dr. Lamar stated in the *Journal of the American Geriatric Society* (Vol. XIV, No. 3, 1966):

"The physical rehabilitation and enjoyment of living experienced by these patients would seem impossible to match through any other available therapeutic procedure."

UNIVERSAL NEED FOR CHELATION THERAPY

As early as 1968, Dr. Lamar predicted, "I have little doubt that eventually new ligands (chelating agents) will be created that will be effective by the oral route. That will be the big step that will bring chelation therapy of calcium to the reach of any patient suffering from any form of calcific disease.

"The great advance in preventive medicine lies in clearing the arteries of deposits which close them BEFORE the symptoms or attack which makes the disorder obvious to everybody," Dr. Evers declared. "This is where chelation therapy has its greatest future."

The list is growing of Chelation Clinics in America and around the world. In America, contact Dr. Bruce Halstead at 22807 Barton Rd., Grand Terrace, Calif. 92324, phone (714) 783-2773; or write the American College of Advancement in Medicine, 23121 Verdugo Dr. #204, Laguna Hills, CA 92653, phone (800) 532-3688; in California phone (714) 583-7666.

In Europe, contact world famous Dr. Claus Martin, who has the vision, wisdom and education to direct his Four Seasons Clinic in the Bavarian Alps where he gives his chelation, oxygen and life cell therapy. These are remarkable, life-prolonging treatments that will help reverse age-related and cardio-vascular degenerative diseases. Hollywood Stars, Famous Statesmen, etc., have reaped the benefits of his Clinic. There are more than 150 Chelation Clinics in Europe. Write or call Dr. Claus Martin, M.D., Box 244, D-8022 Rottach-Egern, Germany. Phone: 49-8022-26780; FAX 49-8022-24740.

Many people go throughout life committing partial suicide — destroying their health, youth, beauty, talents, energies, creative qualities. Indeed, to learn how to be good to oneself is often more difficult than to learn how to be good to others.
—Paul C. Bragg

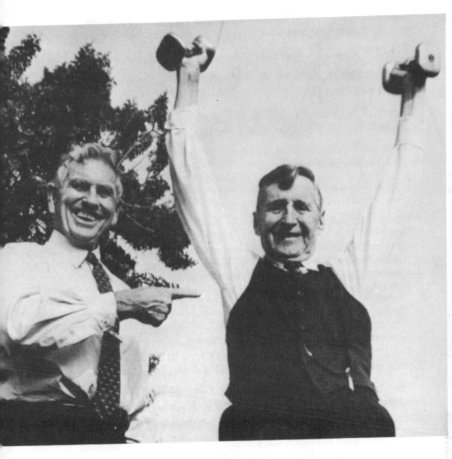

**Paul Bragg with his friend Roy D. White, 106 years young.
They are both keeping fit, healthy and active
living the good health life!**

Our sincere blessings to you dear friends, who make our lives so
worthwhile and fulfilled by reading our teachings on natural living as
our Creator laid down for us all to follow ... Yes—he wants us all to
follow the simple path of natural living and this is what we teach in
our books and health crusades world-wide. Our prayers reach out to
you for the best in health and happiness for you and your loved ones.
This is the birthright He gives us all ... but we must follow the laws
He has laid down for us, so we can reap this precious health,
physically, mentally and spiritually!

Paul C. Bragg

Your healing shall spring up speedily.
--Isaiah 58:8

We Admire Everyone Who Exercises & Keeps Healthy & Fit . . .

IRON-PUMPING OLDSTERS (86 to 96) TRIPLE
THEIR MUSCLE STRENGTH IN 1990 US GOV STUDY

WASHINGTON, June 13, 1990 – Aging nursing home residents, in Boston study, "pumping iron"?

Elderly weight-lifters tripling and quadrupling their muscle strength? Is it possible? Most people would doubt? and wonder?

Government experts on aging gave those questions a resounding "yes" with the results of a new study.

They turned a group of frail Boston nursing-home residents, aged 86 to 96, into weight-lifters to demonstrate that it is never too late to reverse age-related declines in muscle strength. The group participated in a regimen of high-intensity weight-training in a study conducted by the Agriculture Department's Human Nutrition Research Center on Aging at Tufts Unversity in Boston. "A high-intensity weight training program is capable of inducing dramatic increases in muscle strength in frail men and women up to 96 years of age," reported Dr. Maria A. Fiatarone, who headed the study.

AMAZING RESULTS IN 8 WEEKS

"The favorable response to strength training in our subjects was remarkable in light of their very advanced age, extremely sedentary habits, multiple chronic diseases and functional disabilities and nutritional inadequacies.

The elderly weight-lifters increased their muscle strength by anywhere from three-fold to four-fold in as little as eight weeks. Fiatarone said they probably were stronger at the end of the program than they had been in years!

Fiatarone and her associates emphasized the safety of such a closely supervised weight-lifting program, even among people in frail health. The average age of the 10 participants, for instance, was 90. Six had coronary heart disease; seven had arthritis; six had bone fractures resulting from osteoporosis; four had high blood pressure; & all had been physcially inactive for years. Yet no serious medical problems resulted from the program.

A few of the participants did report minor muscle and joint aches, but nine of the 10 completed the program. One man, aged 86, felt a pulling sensation at the site of a previous hernia incision and dropped out after four weeks.

The study participants, drawn from a 712-bed long-term care facility in Boston, worked out three times a week. They performed three sets of eight repetitions with each leg on a weight-lifting machine. The weights were gradually increased from about 10 pounds initially to about 40 pounds at the end of the eight-week program.

Fiatarone said the study carries potentially important implications for older people, who represent a growing proportion of the population. A decline in muscle strength and size is one of the more predictable features of aging.

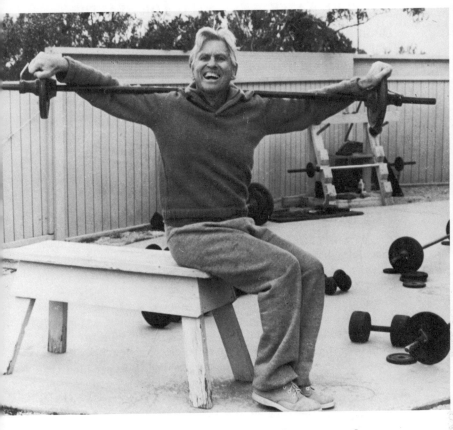

Paul Bragg lifts weights three times a week.

Muscle strength in the average adult decreases by 30 percent to 50 percent during the course of life. Experts on aging do not know whether the decrease is an unavoidable consequence of aging or results mainly from sedentary lifestyle and other controlable factors.

Muscle atrophy and weakness is not merely a cosmetic problem in elderly people, especially the frail elderly. Researchers have linked muscle weakness with recurrent falls, a major cause of immobility and death in the American elderly population. This is causing millions of dollars yearly in staggering medical costs.

Previous studies have suggested that weight training can be helpful in reversing age-related muscle weakness. But Fiatarone said physicians have been reluctant to recommend weight-lifting for frail elderly with multiple health problems. This new government study might be changing their minds. Also, this study shows the great importance of keeping the 640 body muscles as active and fit as possible to maintain general good health.

PURE WATER — ESSENTIAL FOR HEALTH!

Distilled water is one of the world's best and purest waters! It is excellent for detoxification and fasting programs and for helping clean out all the cells, organs, and fluids of the body because it can help carry away so many harmful substances!

Water from chemically-treated public water systems and even from many wells and springs is likely to be loaded with poisonous chemicals and toxic trace elements.

Depending upon the kind of piping that the water has been run through, the water in our homes, offices, schools, hospitals, etc., is likely to be overloaded with zinc (from old-fashioned galvanized pipes) or with copper and cadmium (from copper pipes). These trace elements are released in excessive quantity by the chemical action of the water on the metals of the water pipes.

Yes, pure water is essential for health, either from the natural juices of vegetables, fruits, and other foods, or from the water of high purity obtained by steam distillation which is the best method, or by one of the new high-efficiency deionization processes.

The body is constantly working for you . . . breaking down old bone and tissue cells and replacing them with new ones. As the body casts off the old minerals and other products of broken-down cells, it must obtain new supplies of the essential elements for the new cells. Moreover, Scientists are only now beginning to understand that various kinds of dental problems, different types of arthritis, and even some forms of hardening of the arteries are due to varying kinds of imbalances in the levels of calcium, phosphorus, and magnesium in the body. Disorders can also be caused by imbalances in the ratios of various minerals to each other.

Each individual healthy body requires a proper balance within itself of all the nutritive elements. It is just as bad for any individual to have too much of one item as it is to have too little of that one or of another one. It takes appropriate levels of phosphorus and magnesium to keep calcium in solution so it can be formed into new cells of bone and teeth. Yet, there must not be too much of those nor too little calcium in the diet, or old bone will be taken away but new bone will not be formed.

In addition, we now know that diets which are unbalanced and inappropriate for a given individual can deplete the body of calcium, magnesium, potassium, and other major and minor elements.

Diets which are high in meats, fish, eggs, grains, nuts, seeds, or their products may provide unbalanced excesses of phosphorus which will deplete calcium and magnesium from the bones and tissues of the body and cause them to be lost in the urine.

A diet high in fats will tend to increase the uptake of phosphorus from the intestines relative to calcium and other basic minerals. Such a high-fat diet can produce losses of calcium, magnesium, and other basic minerals in the same way a high-phosphorus diet does.

Diets excessively high in fruits or their juices may provide unbalanced excesses of potassium in the body, and calcium and magnesium will again be lost from the body through the urine.

Deficiencies of calcium and magnesium . . . for example can produce all kinds of problems in the body ranging from dental decay and osteoporosis to muscular cramping, hyper-activity, muscular twitching, poor sleep patterns, and excessive frequency of uncontrolled patterns of urination. Similarly, deficiencies of other minerals, or imbalances in the levels of those minerals, can produce many other problems in the body.

Therefore, it is important to clean and detoxify the body through fasting and through using distilled or other pure water as well as healthy organically-grown vegetable and fruit juices. At the same time, it is also important to provide the body with adequate sources of new minerals. This can be done by eating a widely-distributed diet of wholesome vegetables, including kelp and other sea vegetables for adults and healthy mother's milk for infants, and certified raw goat's or cow's milk for those children and adults who are not adversely affected by milk products . . . but most processed home homogenized milks we do not suggest using.

But, despite dietary sources such as these, many adults and children in so-called civilized cultures will be found to have low levels of essential minerals in their bodies due to losses caused by coffee, tea, carbonated beverages, and long-term bad diets containing too much sugar and other sweets as well as products made from refined flours and containing refined table salt.

In addition, the body's organ systems can be thrown out of balance by continuing stress, by toxins in our air and water, by disease-produced injuries, and by pre-natal deficiencies in the mother's diet or life style.

As a result, many, if not most people in our so-called civilization may need to take mineral supplements such as the new chelated multiple mineral preparations as well as a broad-range multiple-vitamin tablet.

BORON – MIRACLE TRACE MINERAL FOR HEALTHY BONES

BORON – Trace mineral for healthy bones helps the body have more Calcium, Mineral & Hormones! Boron is found in vegetables, fruits, nut and especially good sources are broccoli, prunes, dates, raisins, almonds, peanuts and soybeans.

PURE WATER (H²O) A PRIME REQUISITE OF HEALT[

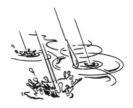

THE 65% WATERY HUMAN

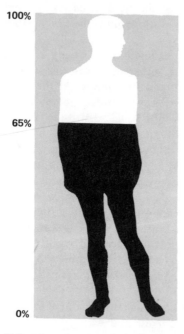

100%

65%

0%

THE 65% WATERY HUMAN

The amount of water in the human body, averaging 65 per cent, varies considerably from person to person and even from one part of the body to another (right). A lean man may have as much as 70 per cent of his weight in the form of body water, while a woman, because of her larger proportion of water-poor fatty tissues, may be only 52 per cent water. The lowering of the water content in the blood is what triggers the hypothalamus, the brain's thirst center to send out its familiar demand for a drink.

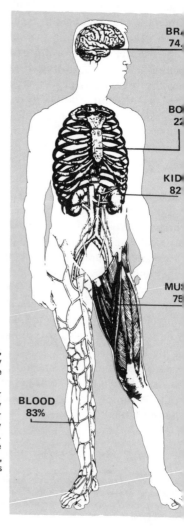

BR
74.

BO
22

KID
82

MU
75

BLOOD
83%

"Water Is The Best Drink For A Wise Man" — Henry Thoreau

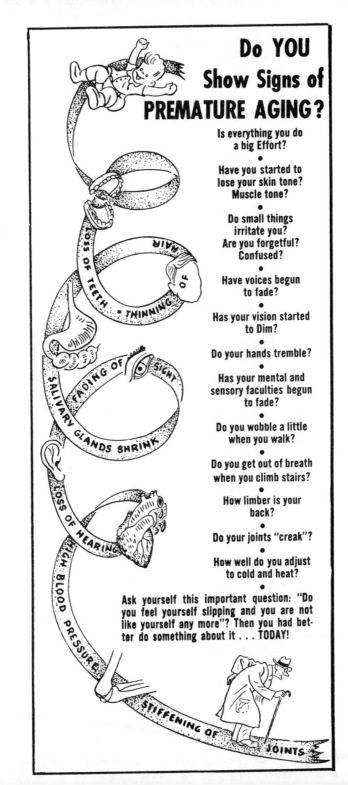

Do YOU Show Signs of PREMATURE AGING?

Is everything you do a big Effort?

•

Have you started to lose your skin tone? Muscle tone?

•

Do small things irritate you? Are you forgetful? Confused?

•

Have voices begun to fade?

•

Has your vision started to Dim?

•

Do your hands tremble?

•

Has your mental and sensory faculties begun to fade?

•

Do you wobble a little when you walk?

•

Do you get out of breath when you climb stairs?

•

How limber is your back?

•

Do your joints "creak"?

•

How well do you adjust to cold and heat?

•

Ask yourself this important question: "Do you feel yourself slipping and you are not like yourself any more"? Then you had better do something about it ... TODAY!

Take time
for **12** things

1 **Take time to Work—**
   it is the price of success.

2 **Take time to Think—**
   it is the source of power.

3 **Take time to Play—**
   it is the secret of youth.

4 **Take time to Read—**
   it is the foundation of knowledge.

5 **Take time to Worship—**
   it is the highway of reverance and washes the
   dust of earth from our eyes.

6 **Take time to Help and Enjoy Friends—**
   it is the source of happiness.

7 **Take time to Love—**
   it is the one sacrament of life.

8 **Take time to Dream—**
   it hitches the soul to the stars.

9 **Take time to Laugh—**
   it is the singing that helps with life's loads.

10 **Take time for Beauty—**
   it is everywhere in nature.

11 **Take time for Health—**
   it is the true wealth and treasure of life.

12 **Take time to Plan—**
   it is the secret of being able to have time to
   take time for the first eleven things.

From the Bragg home to your home we share our years of health knowledge—years of living close to God and Nature and what joys of fruitful, radiant living this produces—this my Father and I share with you and your loved ones.

With blessings for Health and Happiness,

Patricia Bragg

3 John:2 My dear friend, I pray that everything may go well with you, and that you may be in good health—as I know you are well in spirit.

Morning Resolve

I will this day live a simple, sincere and serene life, repelling promptly every thought of impurity, discontent, anxiety, discouragement and self-seeking. I will cultivate cheerfulness, happiness, charity and the love of brotherhood; exercising economy in expenditure, generosity in giving, carefulness in conversation and diligence in appointed service. I pledge fidelity to every trust and a childlike faith in God, in particular, I will be faithful in those habits of prayer, study, work, physical exercise, deep breathing and good posture. I shall fast one 24 hour period each week, eat only natural foods and get sufficient sleep each night. I will make every effort to improve myself physically, mentally and spiritually every day.

Morning prayer used by Paul C. Bragg and Patricia Bragg

WE THANK THEE

For flowers that bloom about our feet;
   For song of bird and hum of bee;
For all things fair we hear or see,
   Father in heaven we thank Thee!
For blue of stream and blue of sky;
   For pleasant shade of branches high;
For fragrant air and cooling breeze;
   For beauty of the blooming trees,
Father in heaven, we thank Thee!
   For mother-love and father-care,
For brothers strong and sisters fair;
   For love at home and here each day;
For guidance lest we go astray,
   Father in heaven, we thank Thee!
For this new morning with its light;
   For rest and shelter of the night;
For health and food, for love and friends;
   For every thing His goodness sends,
Father in heaven, we thank Thee!

- Ralph Waldo Emerson

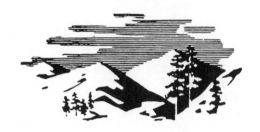

TEN HEALTH COMMANDMENTS

Thou shall respect the body as the highest manifestation of life.

Thou shall abstain from all unnatural, devitalized food and stimulating beverages.

Thou shall nourish thy body with only Natural unprocessed, "live" food, - that . . .

Thou shall extend the years in health for loving, charitable service.

Thou shall regenerate thy body by the right balance of activity and rest.

Thou shall purify thy cells, tissue and blood with pure fresh air and sunshine.

Thou shall abstain from ALL food when out of sorts in mind or body.

Thou shall keep thy thoughts, words and emotions, pure, calm and uplifting.

Thou shall increase thy knowledge of Nature's laws, abide therewith, and enjoy the fruits of thy life's labor.

Thou shall lift up thyself and thy brother man with thine own obedience to God's Natural, Pure Laws of Living.

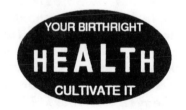

YOUR BIRTHRIGHT

HEALTH

CULTIVATE IT

---

*"Teach me Thy way, O Lord;
and Lead me in a plain path . . . "*
Psalms 97:11

SEND FOR IMPORTANT
FREE
HEALTH BULLETINS

Let Patricia Bragg send you, your relatives and friends the latest News Bulletins on Health and Nutrition Discoveries. These are sent periodically. Please enclose two stamps for each U.S.A. name listed. Foreign listings send international postal reply coupons. Please print or type addresses, thank you.

HEALTH SCIENCE Box 7, Santa Barbara, California 93102 U.S.A.

● _____

Name

_____ ( ) _____

Address   Phone

_____

City   State   Zip Code

- -

● _____

Name

_____ ( ) _____

Address   Phone

_____

City   State   Zip Code

- -

● _____

Name

_____ ( ) _____

Address   Phone

_____

City   State   Zip Code

- -

● _____

Name

_____ ( ) _____

Address   Phone

_____

City   State   Zip Code

- -

● _____

Name

_____ ( ) _____

Address   Phone

_____

City   State   Zip Code

BRAGG "HOW-TO, SELF HEALTH" BOO
Authored by America's First Family of Hea
Live Longer – Healthier – Stronger Self-Improvement

Qty.	Bragg Book Titles Order Form Health Science ISBN 0-87790	Price
____	**Vegetarian** Gourmet Health **Recipes** (no salt, no sugar, yet delicious)	7.95
____	Bragg's Complete **Gourmet Recipes** for Vital Health—448 pages	8.95
____	The **Miracle of Fasting** (Bragg Bible of Health for physical rejuvenation)	6.95
____	Bragg **Health & Fitness Manual** for All Ages—Swim-Bike-Run	
	A Must for Athletes, Triathletes & Would-Be-Athletes—600 pages	*16.95
____	Build Powerful **Nerve Force** (reduce stress, fear, anger, worry)	5.95
____	Keep Your **Heart** & Cardio-Vascular System Healthy & Fit at Any Age	5.95
____	The Natural Way to **Reduce** (lose 10 pounds in 10 days)	5.95
____	The Shocking Truth About **Water** (learn safest water to drink & why)	5.95
____	Your Health and Your **Hair**, Nature's Way to Beautiful Hair (easy-to-do method)	5.95
____	**Healthful Eating** Without Confusion (removes doubt & questions)	5.95
____	Salt-Free Raw **Sauerkraut Recipes** (learn to make your own)	2.95
____	Nature's Healing System to Improve **Eyesight** in 90 days (foods, exercises, etc.)	5.95
____	Super Brain **Breathing** for Super Health & High Energy (can double your energy)	3.95
____	Building Strong **Feet** — Complete Program	5.95
____	**Toxicless Diet**-Purification & Healing System (Stay Ageless Program)	3.95
____	Powerful Health Uses of **Apple Cider Vinegar** (how to live active to 120)	3.95
____	**Fitness/Spine Motion** – For More Flexible, Pain-free Back	3.95
____	Building **Health & Youthfulness**	1.75
____	**Nature's Way** to Health (simple method for long, healthy life)	3.95
____	The Philosophy of **Super Health**	1.75
____	**South Sea Abdomen Culture** for Perfect Elimination & Trim Waist	1.75

Total Copies	Prices subject to change without notice.	TOTAL BOOKS	$

**Shipping: Please add $1.50 for first book and
75¢ each additional or $3.00 each for airmail**

*Add $3.00 shipping for each Bragg Fitness Manual
U.S. retail book orders over $20 add $3.00 only

Please Specify:

☐ Check ☐ Money Order ☐ Cash ☐ Credit Card

Charge My Order To: ☐ Visa ☐ MasterCard

Shipping & Handling	
Ca. Residents add sales tax	
TOTAL ENCLOSED $	

Please U.S. funds only

Credit Card
Number: __ __ __ __ — __ __ __ __ — __ __ __ __ — __   Card Expires: __

[MasterCard] [VISA] Signature: _____

CREDIT CARD
CUSTOMERS ONLY
USE OUR
FAST ORDER SERVICE:
(800)-446-1990

In a hurry? Call (805) 968-1020. We can accept N
or VISA phone orders only. Please prepare your orde
order form. It will speed your call & serve as your or
Hours: 9 to 4pm Pacific Time, Monday to Thursday . . .
fax your order: **FAX (805) 968-1001.**

Mail to: **HEALTH SCIENCE, Box 7, Santa Barbara, CA 93102 U**

Please Print or Type – Be sure to give street & house number to facilitate delive

Name _____

Address _____   Apt. No. _____

City _____   State _____

(___) _____
Phone   Zip __ __ __ __ __

Order your Bragg Health Books Today – For a Healthier To

SEND FOR IMPORTANT FREE HEALTH BULLETINS

Let Patricia Bragg send you, your relatives and friends the latest News Bulletins on Health and Nutrition Discoveries. These are sent periodically. Please enclose two stamps for each U.S.A. name listed. Foreign listings send international postal reply coupons. Please print or type addresses, thank you.

HEALTH SCIENCE Box 7, Santa Barbara, California 93102 U.S.A.

●
_____
Name

_____( )_____
Address   Phone

_____
City   State   Zip Code

- -

●
_____
Name

_____( )_____
Address   Phone

_____
City   State   Zip Code

- -

●
_____
Name

_____( )_____
Address   Phone

_____
City   State   Zip Code

- -

●
_____
Name

_____( )_____
Address   Phone

_____
City   State   Zip Code

- -

●
_____
Name

_____( )_____
Address   Phone

_____
City   State   Zip Code

BRAGG "HOW-TO, SELF HEALTH" BOOKS
Authored by America's First Family of Health
Live Longer – Healthier – Stronger Self-Improvement Libra

Qty.	Bragg Book Titles Order Form Health Science ISBN 0-87790	Price	Total
____	**Vegetarian** Gourmet Health **Recipes** (no salt, no sugar, yet delicious)	7.95	
____	Bragg's Complete **Gourmet Recipes** for Vital Health—448 pages	8.95	
____	The **Miracle of Fasting** (Bragg Bible of Health for physical rejuvenation)	6.95	
____	Bragg **Health & Fitness Manual** for All Ages—Swim-Bike-Run		
	A Must for Athletes, Triathletes & Would-Be-Athletes—600 pages	*16.95	
____	Build Powerful **Nerve Force** (reduce stress, fear, anger, worry)	5.95	
____	Keep Your **Heart** & Cardio-Vascular System Healthy & Fit at Any Age	5.95	
____	The Natural Way to **Reduce** (lose 10 pounds in 10 days)	5.95	
____	The Shocking Truth About **Water** (learn safest water to drink & why)	5.95	
____	Your Health and Your **Hair**, Nature's Way to Beautiful Hair (easy-to-do method) .	5.95	
____	**Healthful Eating** Without Confusion (removes doubt & questions)	5.95	
____	Salt-Free Raw **Sauerkraut Recipes** (learn to make your own)	2.95	
____	Nature's Healing System to Improve **Eyesight** in 90 days (foods, exercises, etc.)	5.95	
____	Super Brain **Breathing** for Super Health & High Energy (can double your energy)	3.95	
____	Building Strong **Feet** — Complete Program	5.95	
____	**Toxicless Diet**-Purification & Healing System (Stay Ageless Program)	3.95	
____	Powerful Health Uses of **Apple Cider Vinegar** (how to live active to 120)	3.95	
____	**Fitness/Spine Motion** – For More Flexible, Pain-free Back	3.95	
____	Building **Health & Youthfulness**	1.75	
____	**Nature's Way** to Health (simple method for long, healthy life)	3.95	
____	The Philosophy of **Super Health**	1.75	
____	**South Sea Abdomen Culture** for Perfect Elimination & Trim Waist	1.75	

Total Copies	Prices subject to change without notice.	TOTAL BOOKS	$

Shipping: Please add $1.50 for first book and
75¢ each additional or $3.00 each for airmail

	Shipping & Handling	

*Add $3.00 shipping for each Bragg Fitness Manual
U.S. retail book orders over $20 add $3.00 only

	Ca. Residents add sales tax	

Please Specify:

	TOTAL ENCLOSED $	

☐ Check ☐ Money Order ☐ Cash ☐ Credit Card

Please U.S. funds only

Charge My Order To: ☐ Visa ☐ MasterCard

month   ye

Credit Card
Number: _ _ _ _ _ _ _ _ _ _ _ _ _ _ _ _   Card Expires: |

[MasterCard] [VISA] Signature: _____

In a hurry? Call (805) 968-1020. We can accept MasterC
or VISA phone orders only. Please prepare your order using
order form. It will speed your call & serve as your order rec
Hours: 9 to 4pm Pacific Time, Monday to Thursday ... or you
fax your order: **FAX (805) 968-1001.**

Mail to: **HEALTH SCIENCE, Box 7, Santa Barbara, CA 93102 U.S.A**

<u>Please Print or Type</u> – Be sure to give street & house number to facilitate delivery BOF-

Name _____

Address _____   Apt. No. _____

City _____   State _____

(____) _____   Zip _ _ _ _ _
Phone

Order your Bragg Health Books Today – For a Healthier Tomorr

SEND FOR IMPORTANT
FREE
HEALTH BULLETINS

Let Patricia Bragg send you, your relatives and friends the latest
News Bulletins on Health and Nutrition Discoveries. These are
sent periodically. Please enclose two stamps for each U.S.A.
name listed. Foreign listings send international postal reply
coupons. Please print or type addresses, thank you.

HEALTH SCIENCE Box 7, Santa Barbara, California 93102 U.S.A.

●
_____
Name

_____( )_____
Address   Phone

_____
City   State   Zip Code

●
_____
Name

_____( )_____
Address   Phone

_____
City   State   Zip Code

●
_____
Name

_____( )_____
Address   Phone

_____
City   State   Zip Code

●
_____
Name

_____( )_____
Address   Phone

_____
City   State   Zip Code

●
_____
Name

_____( )_____
Address   Phone

_____
City   State   Zip Code

BRAGG ALL NATURAL LIQUID AMINOS
Order Form

Delicious, Healthy Alternative to Tamari-Soy Sauce

BRAGG LIQUID AMINOS — Nutrition you need...taste you will love...a family favorite over 75 years. A delicious source of nutritious life-renewing protein from soybeans on Add to or spray over casseroles, soups, sauces, gravies, potatoes, popcorn, a vegetables. An ideal "pick-me-up" broth at work, home or the gym. Gourmet hea replacement for Tamari & Soy Sauce. Start today and add more Amino Acids for healt living to your daily diet — the easy BRAGG LIQUID AMINOS Way!

DASH or SPRAY for NEW TASTE DELIGHTS! PROVEN & ENJOYED BY MILLIONS.

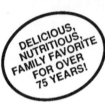

DELICIOUS, NUTRITIOUS, FAMILY FAVORITE FOR OVER 75 YEARS!

Dash of Bragg Aminos Brings New Taste Delights to Season:

- Salads
- Dressings
- Soups
- Vegies
- Rice/Beans
- Tofu
- Tempeh
- Wok foods
- Stir-frys
- Casseroles & Potatoes
- Meats
- Poultry
- Fish
- Popcorn
- Gravies
- Sauces
- Macrobiotics

Pure Soybeans and Pure Water Only

- No Added Sodium
- No Coloring Agents
- No Preservatives
- Not Fermented
- No Chemicals
- No Additives
- No MSG

BRAGG LIQUID AMINOS

SIZE	PRICE	SHIPPING	AMT.	TOTAL $
16 oz.	$ 3.95 ea.	Please add $3.00 for 1st bottle/$1.50 for each additional bottle		.
32 oz.	$ 6.45 ea.	Please add $3.90 for 1st bottle/$1.90 for each additional bottle		.
16 oz.	$ 47.40 ea.	Case/12 bottles add $9.00 per case		.
32 oz.	$ 77.40 ea.	Case/12 bottles add $14.00 per case		.

Total Aminos	$
Shipping & Handling	.
Total Enclosed	$.

Please Specify: (U.S. Funds Only)

☐ Check   ☐ Money Order   ☐ Cash   ☐ Credit Card

Charge My Order To: ☐ Visa   ☐ MasterCard

Credit Card
Number: _ _ _ _ _ _ _ _ _ _ _ _ _ _ _ _   Card Expires: ___ | Month Ye___

MasterCard   *VISA*   Signature:_____

CREDIT CARD CUSTOMERS ONLY USE OUR FAST PHONE SERVICE: (800) 446-1990

In a hurry? Call (805) 968-1028. We can accept MasterCar VISA phone orders only. Please prepare your order using tl order form. It will speed your call & serve as your order reco Hours: 9 to 4 pm Pacific Time, Monday to Thursday ... or you c fax your order to: **FAX (805) 968-1001.**

Mail to: **HEALTH SCIENCE, Box 7, Santa Barbara, CA 93102 USA**

Please Print or Type – Be sure to give street & house number to facilitate delivery

A-BOF-

Name _____

Address _____   Apt. No. _____

City _____   State _____

(_____) _____

Phone

Zip _ _ _ _ _

Bragg Aminos —Taste You Love, Nutrition You Need

PATRICIA BRAGG N.D., Ph.D.
Angel of Health & Healing
Lecturer, Author, Nutritionist, Health Educator & Fitness Advisor to World Leaders, Glamorous Hollywood Stars, Singers, Dancers & Athletes.

Daughter of the world renowned health authority, Paul C. Bragg, Patricia Bragg has won international fame on her own in this field. She conducts Health and Fitness Seminars for Women's, Men's, Youth and Church Groups throughout the world... and promotes Bragg "How-To, Self-Health" Books in Lectures, on Radio and Television Talk Shows throughout the English-speaking world. Consultants to Presidents and Royalty, to the Stars of Stage, Screen and TV and to Champion Athletes, Patricia Bragg and her father are Co-Authors of the Bragg Health Library of Instructive, Inspiring Books that promote a healthy lifestyle for a long, vital, active life!

Patricia herself is the symbol of perpetual youth and super energy. She is a living and sparkling example of her and her father's healthy lifestyle precepts and this she shares world-wide.

A fifth generation Californian on her mother's side, Patricia was reared by the Natural Health Method from infancy. In school, she not only excelled in athletics but also won high honors in her studies and her counseling. She is an accomplished musician and dancer... as well as tennis player, swimmer and mountain climber... and the youngest woman ever to be granted a U.S. Patent. Patricia is a popular gifted Health Teacher and a dynamic, in-demand Talk Show Guest where she spreads simple, easy-to-follow health teachings for everyone.

Man's body is the Temple of the Holy Spirit, and our creator wants us filled with Joy and Health for a long walk with Him for Eternity. The Bragg Crusade of Health and Fitness (3 John 2) has carried her around the world... spreading physical, spiritual, emotional and mental health and joy. Health is our birthright and Patricia teaches how to prevent the destruction of our health from man-made wrong habits of living.

Patricia's been Health Consultant to American Presidents and to the British Royal Family, to Betty Cuthbert, Australia's "Golden Girl" who holds 16 world records and four Olympic gold medals in women's track and to New Zealand's Olympic Track Star Allison Roe. Among those who come to her for advice are some of Hollywood's top stars from Clint Eastwood to the ever youthful singing group The Beach Boys and their families, singing stars of the Metropolitan Opera and top ballet stars. Patricia's message is of world-wide appeal to the people of all ages, nationalities and walks-of-life. Those who follow the Bragg Health Books & attend the Bragg Crusades are living testimonials like Super Athlete, Ageless - Jack LaLanne—at age 14 he went from sickness to health.

Patricia Bragg inspires you to Renew, Rejuvenate & Revitalize your life with the "Bragg Healthy Lifestyle" Seminars and Lectures world-wide. These are life-changing and millions have benefited with a longer, healthier life! She would love to share her Crusade with your organizations, businesses, churches, etc. Also, she is a perfect radio and T.V. talk show guest to spread the message of health and fitness in your area.

Write or call for requests and information:
HEALTH SCIENCE, BOX 7, SANTA BARBARA, CA 93102 1-805-968-1028

PAUL C. BRAGG N.D., Ph.D.
Life Extension Specialist • World Health Crusader
Lecturer and Advisor to Olympic Athletes, Royalty, and Stars
Originator of Health Food Stores - Now World-wide

For almost a Century, Living Proof that his
"Health and Fitness Way of Life" Works Wonders!

Paul C. Bragg is the Father of the Health Movement in America. This dynamic Crusader for worldwide health and fitness is responsible for more "firsts" in the history of Health than any other individual. Here are a few of his incredible pioneering achievements that the world now enjoys:

- Bragg originated, named and opened the first "Health Food Store" in America.
- Bragg Crusades pioneered the first Health Lectures across America, inspiring followers to open health stores in cities across the land and now world-wide.
- Bragg introduced pineapple juice and tomato juice to the American public.
- He was the first to introduce and distribute honey nationwide.
- He introduced Juice Therapy in America by importing the first hand-juicers.
- Bragg pioneered Radio Health Programs from Hollywood three times daily. Paul and Patricia pioneered a Health TV show from Hollywood to spread "Health and Happiness"... the name of the show! It included exercises, health recipes, visual demonstrations, and guest appearances of famous, health-minded people.
- He created the first health foods & products and made them available nation-wide: herb teas, health beverages, seven-grain cereals and crackers, health cosmetics, health candies, vitamins and mineral supplements, wheat germ, digestive enzymes from papaya, herbs & kelp seasonings, amino acids from soybeans. He inspired others to follow and now thousands of health items are available worldwide.
- He opened the first health restaurants and health spas in America.

Crippled by TB as a teenager, Bragg developed his own eating, breathing and exercising program to rebuild his body into an ageless, tireless, painfree citadel of glowing, radiant health. He excelled in running, swimming, biking, progressive weight training, and mountain-climbing. He made an early pledge to God, in return for his renewed health, to spend the rest of his life showing others the road to health... Paul Bragg made good his pledge!

A living legend and beloved counselor to millions, Bragg was the inspiration and personal advisor on diet and fitness to top Olympic Stars from 4-time swimming Gold Medalist Murray Rose to 3-time track Gold Medalist Betty Cuthbert of Australia, his relative Don Bragg (pole-vaulting Gold Medalist), and countless others. Jack LaLanne, "the original TV King of Fitness," says, "Bragg saved my life at age 14 when I attended the Bragg Crusade in Oakland, California." From the earliest days, Bragg was advisor to the greatest Hollywood Stars, and to giants of American Business. J. C. Penney, Del E. Webb, and Conrad Hilton are just a few that he inspired to long, successful, healthy, active lives!

Dr. Bragg changed the lives of millions worldwide in all walks of life... through his Health Crusades, Books, Tapes and Radio, TV and personal appearances.

HEALTH SCIENCE Box 7, Santa Barbara, California 93102 U.S.A.